CANCER

A Threat To Your Life ?

or

A Chance To Take Control Of Your Future ?

CANCER A Threat To Your Life? **or** A Chance To Control Your Future

First published 2006

ISBN 0-473-11327-9

DESIGNED & PRINTED IN NEW ZEALAND BY LIFEWAY PRINT LTD info@lifeway.co.nz

PUBLISHED BY LEWIS PUBLICATIONS PO BOX 27871 MT ROSKILL AUCKLAND

The Choice Is Yours!

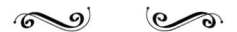

Over the years, Drs Gerald and Monica Lewis have developed a special interest in helping people who have developed cancer. They both graduated from Otago Medical School, New Zealand in 1968, and after a few years of practice, both came to realise the limitations of conventional medical treatments - surgery, drugs and radiotherapy - and so have introduced many complementary treatments into their practice.

Monica is a general practitioner (family practitioner) who has specialised in counseling and helping people with more complex conditions for whom conventional health services have little more to offer. She has included nutritional medicine, the use of bio-identical hormones and mind/body medicine into her routine medical therapies.

Gerald finished his postgraduate training in the United Kingdom where he specialised in general medicine and cardiology. He was awarded his Doctorate of Medicine (MD) and, for discoveries he made in the treatment of high blood pressure, he has been cited in both Who's Who in the World and Who's Who in Medicine.

As part of his medical practice, he has been treating patients with cancer for most of his career, but in the last few years, working at the Centre for Advanced Medicine in Auckland, his interest in cancer has deepened. This is especially so when treating patients where their medical advisors feel they have reached the end of the line with conventional treatments. Intravenous high dose vitamin C is one very powerful therapy which he has been offering to cancer patients, hopefully to extend life, but also, and most important, to improve the quality of life and reduce discomfort.

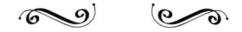

Why We Have Written This Book

In our experience, when a person is told they have cancer, usually their mind becomes confused and their thinking goes into turmoil. It is hard to think clearly and the amount of information available from many sources - well meaning friends, books, the internet, health professionals and alternative practitioners - is usually overwhelming and may also be conflicting. Unfortunately many of the treatments are very costly.

"We have realised that with our combined medical experience of almost 80 years, we are probably in a better situation to sift through this confusing and sometimes contradictory information.

We have written this book for our patients and for any other people who have cancer themselves, or who have friends or relatives with the disease. We want to make this information available to as many people as possible. Please feel free to copy sections to give to friends if you wish but because many of the sections are inter-related it is best to review the whole book.

We are also producing a 'talking book' on CD for people who find it difficult to read."

We hope you find this book helpful and informative. We would welcome feed back for subsequent printings.

(Email glewis@clear.net.nz)

B Monica Lewis MB ChB

Gerald R J Lewis MB ChB, FRCP (UK), FRACP, MD (Otago)

~ *We Dedicate This Book To* ~

Our patients, many of whom have become friends and who have inspired us with their fortitude, love, concern for others and strength of resolve to be healed. Their love has taught us so much. Some have been pronounced cured while others wait for us across the divide.

Many people have assisted us in varying ways in the writing, proofing and editing of this book. We are grateful to our 3 daughters Debbie, Susie and Mandy who have pressed us to make time in our busy schedules for what they knew was in our hearts; Dr Hugh Riordan for his advice and inspiration, Victor Marks who first encouraged us to share our thoughts in writing; Sherry Burton for her critical overview and suggestions; Brian Fergusson, who owns the lovely voice reading our talking book version; Andrew Kellett, our proof reader and editor; Choo, David and Jackson; our staff at the Centre for Advanced Medicine who look after our patients – Gay, Steph and Káren, whose positivity and caring are a constant inspiration to us.

We are also indebted to Andriano and Lance of Lifeway Print who made printing this book such a breeze and for their creative suggestions and advice.

And finally to Alan, Simon and Dave.

CONTENTS

PART 1
Dealing With Cancer

CONTENTS

PART 2
Cancer Prevention

Part 1

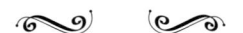

Dealing With Cancer

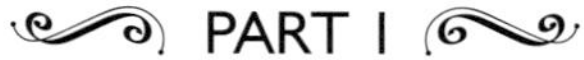

PART I

Dealing With Cancer

INTRODUCTION

In this book, by bringing together most of the therapies available, we aim to enable a person with cancer to plan a therapy pathway with some understanding and confidence.

Up to 90% of people diagnosed with cancer consider using complementary therapies and three quarters do not tell their doctor what they are doing. In this book we want to show the value and usefulness of both conventional and complementary treatments. Armed with this information, we would encourage you to discuss all forms of treatment with all your health providers.

What, Why and When

In this book we will explore -

What **treatments are available**
Why **they work, or theories on why they might work**
When **people with cancer should consider using them**

Cancer can be beaten!

Many people, when told they have cancer believe that this is a death sentence. But with modern treatments this is now far from reality.
Be aware of these facts:

- People have been cured from every type of cancer,
- Cancer is the most curable of all chronic diseases (yes this is true!)
- In the USA alone there are 8 million people living with cancer and 3 million of them are considered cured.

The long term survival rate for people with cancer is far better than most people realise. For all cancers the 20-year survival rate is over 50%, and it is higher in thyroid and testis (90%), melanoma and prostate (80%) bladder and Hodgkin's (70%), breast (65%) and cervix (60%).

More than half of all people with bowel, rectal, ovarian and kidney cancer live for more than 20 years. [1]

With the volume of research being done world wide, we are confident that within 20 years we will almost certainly have beaten cancer (in the same way that previous generations have beaten bacterial and viral infections.)

It is essential to feel positive towards your body and your health, because with cancer, more than with any other disease, our attitude of mind towards the illness and the strength of our resolve to recover, is in most cases more important than any other treatment.

Our attitude to the illness and the strength of our resolve to recover is probably more important than any other treatment.

What is cancer?

Our bodies are made up of trillions of cells, each with a limited life (from days to months). Throughout our life, these cells wear out, and are replaced with new cells. Sometimes the new cells are imperfect; the immune system recognizes these and destroys them, just as it does with invading viruses and bacteria. Cancer develops when cell duplication goes wrong and for some reason the immune system does not destroy the abnormal cells.

These abnormal cancer cells slip through the defense system, grow into a new clump of cells and then start multiplying out of control. In today's toxic world, we all develop these abnormal cells from time to time but the immune system is able to function correctly and destroy them before they proceed to multiply.

Initially the cancer cells grow where they first occurred, but sometimes small clumps can break off and travel in the blood or lymph to other parts of the body and start growing there – these are called metastases or cancer secondaries.

So it seems obvious – the most important way to prevent, arrest and treat cancer is to support the body's immune system. Remember that the immune system is designed to destroy foreign or 'different' cells (like viruses and bacteria) and it also considers cancer cells to be abnormal and tries its utmost to destroy them as well. However the immune system can become overwhelmed by the number of cancer cells. Many of the treatments we discuss in this book aim to strengthen our immunity in *addition* to damaging the cancer cells. Because our immune system is so powerful, cancer should never be considered incurable. As we have stated above – individuals with every type of cancer have been cured!

> *The most important way to prevent, arrest and treat cancer is to support the body's immune system*

The effects of cancer

As the result of the growth of the cancer cells, a number of things can occur:

1. They invade vital organs and damage them. This accounts for only about one quarter of the deaths from cancer.
2. Release of toxins and chemicals from the growing and dying cancer cells can 'poison' the body and affect the function of the liver, kidney or other organs.
3. Suppressed immunity can lead to severe infections such as pneumonia which can be fatal.
4. Weight loss and debilitation – as the cancer cells grow, they consume most of the body's energy and nutrients. 'Starvation' and depletion of essential nutrients suppress the immune system, cause weight loss and exhaustion, and are the cause of almost half of all cancer deaths.
5. Very rarely, the cancer cells can secrete hormones or other products which can cause unusual symptoms (called the non-metastatic manifestations of cancer).
6. Cancer causes emotional, mental and spiritual problems – anger and frustration, unresolved problems from the past, uncertainty

about the meaning of life, what happens after death. Most people have these and other feelings. People are much healthier when these are openly discussed, rather than being bottled up inside. The relationship with family and friends can also become strained. Conversely, it can become a time of real closeness within the family.

Therapies for cancer

The shattering news that a person has cancer often causes numbness and shock, incomprehension, fear and a feeling of impotence. This stress can cause a number of chemical and hormonal changes within the body, rendering any logical thought and decision making difficult. It is very difficult to obtain well researched and logical advice on what steps to take. There is an overwhelming array of treatments available. Do they work? Could they cause harm? Do they interfere with conventional treatment? All this needs to be weighed up before making a decision on what to do.

In this book we will discuss most of the treatments which can be used, both conventional and complementary. We will endeavour to separate the fads and fiction from the proven facts and hope to provide a balanced overview.

We would encourage you to be open with your oncologist or surgeon and confirm that what you are considering does not clash with their treatments, especially radiotherapy or chemotherapy.

At the present time not many treatment providers know about the wide range of available therapies, but as more information becomes available, the separation between complementary and conventional treatment providers is narrowing.

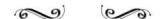

Overview of therapies available to treat cancer

Very rarely is one treatment the 'magic bullet'. But the combined effect of a number of treatments can be extremely powerful and therapeutic. We will start with an overview of possible therapies, then each will be discussed in detail.

1. *A positive attitude towards your illness* is probably the most important factor in successfully overcoming cancer.
   - **a** Develop a good relationship with your doctor of openness and trust
   - **b** Exercise
   - **c** Mental attitude
2. *Cleansing and detoxifying the body.* A clean and unpolluted body, with all its cells free from toxins and poisons, provides a secure foundation - helping the immune system to function at optimum.
   - **a** Bowel cleansing - enemas and colonics
   - **b** Liver detoxification.
   - **c** Eat pure, organic unpolluted food,
   - **d** Drink plenty of clean filtered or pure water.
   - **e** Intravenous heavy metal removal – if there is a history of any exposure
3. *Make the body inhospitable to cancer*
   - **a** Oxygen – cancer cells do not like oxygen,
   - **b** Avoid high blood glucose peaks because cancer cells use glucose as their energy source.
   - **c** Alkaline pH – cancer cells do not like living in an alkaline medium.
   - **d** Reducing the ability of the cancer cells to spread.

4. Strengthen the normal body cells, especially the immune system cells -

- **a** Complete nutrition – high quality food, raw foods, juicing, fruit and cruciferous vegetables.
- **b** Nutritional supplements – high quality supplements to supply what is required and what may be missing
- **c** New therapies which may boost the immune system's fight against cancer.

5. Treatments targeting the cancer cells:

Traditional therapies

- **a** Surgery – removing the tumour, debulking procedures, cryosurgery
- **b** Radiotherapy and brachytherapy
- **c** Chemotherapy
- **d** Hormonal therapies.

Non traditional therapies

- **a** Mind-body medicine
- **b** High dose nutritional supplements
- **c** Herbs
- **d** Intravenous therapies – high dose vitamin C
- **e** Homeopathic therapies and extracts
- **f** Hyperthermia
- **g** Others – magnetic, electric field therapies, live blood and stem cell infusions.....

Now let's study each of these treatments in turn

CHAPTER I

A Positive And Confident Attitude Towards Your Illness

Your health advisors

Your overall treatment plan should be discussed with your main health professional who may be your GP, oncologist or another health practitioner, who should be like the conductor of an orchestra, coordinating your treatment, referring you to other specialists as necessary.

- Make sure he or she is a person you can relate to, who will listen to your opinions and will allow you to have some input into your treatment. Remember this is *your* journey and *you* are ultimately the decision maker.
- If you are unhappy or confused, ask for a second opinion.
- Write down all your questions, perhaps take your partner or a friend with you, take notes and clarify all your questions. Buy a beautiful notebook in which to write all ideas and suggestions, especially the positive ones.
- Find out all the treatment options, their possibility of success, likely side effects and adverse effects. It is your right to know about these so you can weigh up your options. In the past, people accepted treatment and often did not ask about side effects. This knowledge is most important and can affect your decision as to whether to proceed with a treatment.
- If the option you are offered is a major procedure – major surgery, radiotherapy, chemotherapy – if there is doubt in your mind ask if you can have a second opinion just to give you the unreserved conviction that the treatment you are being offered is the best one for you. Ask if the treatment will improve the quality or the length of your life.

Note this does not just apply to conventional medical treatment; if there is some risk or expense involved in a complementary therapy also get a second opinion, but make sure that the person you ask has an complete understanding of the procedure.

- Listen to your oncologist or radiotherapist very carefully. These people are extremely dedicated doctors practicing in what is possibly the most difficult field in medicine. In addition to their years at medical school they have spent many more years undertaking postgraduate training. These people are genuine Specialists spelt with a capital S. Because their training in complementary therapies is limited, like that of most doctors, their understanding of these therapies may be a bit rudimentary. However, their understanding of your cancer and their knowledge of the best and latest therapies using conventional medicine far exceed the information available to any other practitioners. They read the latest journals, attend seminars and conferences – do not ignore their advice.

  In most countries the information overload, financial restrictions and clinical case load placed upon these devoted people makes life very difficult. In addition the personal burden of looking after seriously sick patients (some of whom die) can be utterly draining. For this reason some attempt to cope by retaining a so-called 'clinical detachment' which at times may make them appear a little uncaring. Have no fear, these people care a great deal and they suffer hugely when they lose patients whom in many cases have become personal friends. They need your support almost as much as you require theirs.

As we will discuss below, your confidence that your treatment is going to be of real benefit is possibly the most important part of your healing therapy.

Your attitude and your lifestyle

In most books that discuss how a person can beneficially affect their disease, the most important chapters usually discuss Mind-Body medicine. In the Western world we have forgotten just how much our thoughts, fears and attitudes affect the rest of our body. The Aboriginal bone pointing ceremony shows how powerful the mind can be in a destructive way. Equally, a positive, optimistic, happy attitude can make a huge difference. Those who saw Robin Williams in the Patch Adams movie saw how important caring, happiness and laughter were in helping people to cope with their current situation, and also how it helped their wellbeing and recovery. We encourage you to read some of the many books available.

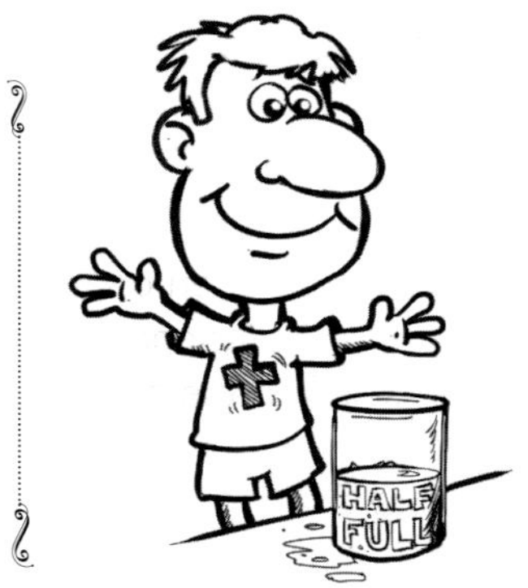

Your mental attitude is probably the most important treatment modality of all. A positive attitude and confidence in your health team, believing that you will recover, is almost essential for a complete healing.

There are many important techniques which can help to achieve this.

- **Meditation** – emptying the mind and creating inner peace is often tremendously helpful. Most non-Western countries practice this and recognise its value. Meditation provides an inner peace and strength and will boost your conviction that you will recover. Read about meditation and attend workshops which are available everywhere. For some notes on about meditation see [Appendix F].
- **Imagery** - for many people this may seem weird, but it really does work. In a meditative state, focus on the immune cells and imagine them moving in like a small army and destroying the cancer cells. Strange though it sounds, it is effective and not just with cancer. Dr Dean Ornish is an American cardiologist who uses imagery in heart patients to open up their arteries. There are many things we don't understand about our minds – some things we just have to take on trust, and this is one of them. Imagery and affirmations link our bodies to the power which created us.
- **Spiritual awareness** and growth are also very important. Whether we acknowledge it or not, we have a dimension as human beings that sets us apart from the animal world. We are a very complex interaction of body, mind and spirit. We may not be aware of the power of our mind

and we often only find out the power of the Spirit in moments of adversity. Almost all cultures acknowledge some greater spiritual force even though it may be expressed in differing ways. Once people realise that their health and wellbeing is in danger, the importance of this spiritual awareness comes into focus. When one becomes ill, it is important to nurture the spiritual side of our existence. This concept is far broader than any one religion. It is linking into the power which created us, with the whole energy of the world, and we can gain strength from it.

- **Be positive** – remember we become and move towards what we focus on. Threfore thinking constantly about cancer, illness and the possibility of dying pulls us down. Think of power and beauty, abundant health and strength, life and love and your mind will move your body in this direction.
- **Ignore any negative comments** from people who should know better. Some people talk about their bad experiences, or criticise conventional or complementary treatments without really knowing about them. Sadly, many doctors do this about vitamins, meditation and other complementary treatments, because they feel that *their* treatment is the only thing which matters. It is important to realise that often their criticisms are made in ignorance with the attitude of "if I don't understand it, then it can't work". If it is doing no harm and the patient believes in it, why knock it?

  A request to all those talking to people with cancer *never, we repeat never criticize or make someone lose faith in a therapy* – providing it is doing no harm. In ways we do not understand, a healthy positive mind strengthens the immune system, and any criticism or attempts to make the patient lose confidence in a therapy, could do them positive harm!

  If it is doing no harm, never criticise or make someone lose faith in a therapy which they believe is doing them good

- **Forgiveness** – always practice forgiveness, do not hold grudges or negative feelings toward others. The only person this is hurting is you. Look at the grievances of the past, study them, forgive the perpetrators (either physically or in your mind), and put the whole experience behind you. This can be a very healing process, because the negative feelings caused by these stresses can actually impair the immune system.

- **Laughter** – people feel better when they laugh because the metabolism is increased and euphoric neurochemicals enter the blood. Laughter has been shown to boost the immune system – it lowers cortisol which enables interleukin 2 and other immune boosters to express themselves. After a session of genuine belly laughing (watching funny movies, Rowan Atkinson, the Goons….) pain can be effectively reduced for many hours.
- **Make your own endorphins** – become your own 'drug factory.' Endorphins are morphine-like 'hormones' created by our bodies to help cope with stress, endure pain and make us feel happy. Long distance runners create endorphins – which enables them to cope better with pain. Any person in distress can also increase their own pain relieving hormones, which can reduce pain, discomfort and depression. [See Appendix E for a list of simple satisfying techniques]

Exercise and lifestyle

Cancer generates feelings of weakness and low energy.

- Walking, especially along a beach or amongst beautiful trees, lifts the spirits, and boosts vitality. Being amid beauty and experiencing the sun, wind and even rain provides a positive spiritual uplift.
- Search out inspiring and moving music, movies and DVDs, books and friends.
- Go out and do things you enjoy, things you have always dreamed of doing.
- Arrange to have a regular massage.

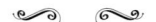

Dr Bernard Fox of Boston University Medical School has described the profile of a person most likely to survive cancer – *"They fought with their doctors, they sought alternative opinions and forms of treatment. They refused to relinquish hope and struggled to survive."*

"Cancers tend to disappear in people who have faith, independence, emotionally transforming experiences, and active involvement in their disease."

In short, people who are really determined to live have a fighting chance to get over the disease.

CHAPTER 2

Detoxifying And Cleansing The Body

Does your body contain toxic levels of heavy metals and other poisons?

In today's world it is almost impossible to avoid fumes, pollution and poisons in air and food. These weaken the body, especially the immune system, and if they are present in high amounts, then it seems logical to consider their removal.

There are some techniques which claim to identify the level of toxins by magnet/electrical and other measurements. Because their mechanism of action is hard to understand within conventional medical thinking, we do not fully understand these and really cannot comment on their accuracy.

Probably the most reliable method is to measure the level of toxins found in the hair, blood or urine. One of the few ways that the body can rid itself of many toxins is through the hair, so the level of heavy metals and other materials found in a properly taken hair sample gives a fairly reliable indication of the current toxic load in the body.

Cleansing and detoxification

Cancer is a toxic disease. The tumour cells often outgrow their blood supply and die. These cells also break down for many other reasons and release toxins into the body causing malaise. Sometimes they can create a noticeable smell. Toxins can also affect healthy body cells and impair their functions. Thus removing toxins is an important add-on to therapy.

- **Drinking plenty of pure, filtered or clean water** – this enables the body to flush more of the toxins out through the kidneys.

Dehydration concentrates the toxins and makes people feel unwell. Everyone should drink at least 8 glasses of water daily, in addition to other drinks. Use water as pure and chemical free as possible.

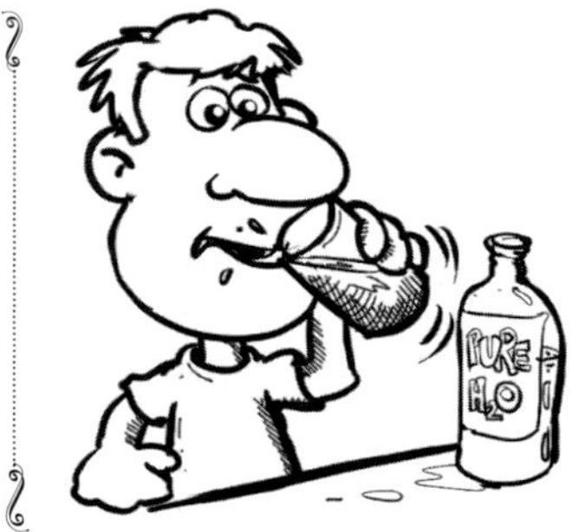

- **Eat quality, unprocessed and organic food** - Trying to rid the body of toxic chemicals and materials is pointless if one continues to eat polluted food which contains toxins, pesticides, fungicides, sprays, heavy metals and poisons. Wash and soak unprocessed food in pure water containing a few drops of ascorbic acid. Eat organic, raw and unprocessed foods as much as possible. Increase your intake of fruit and vegetables, especially sprouted seeds, cruciferous vegetables [see Appendix B] and nuts. Burning and overcooking, especially using hot oils or barbequing, have been shown to increase cancer-inducing chemicals in our food.

- **Eat plenty of fibre in the diet**. Because cancer patients often have a poor appetite this can sometimes be challenging. Fibre is found in fruit and vegetables. There are two types of fibre:

  Soluble fibre - which absorbs toxins and carries them out of the body through the bowel

  Insoluble fibre - which simply keeps the bowels moving, reducing the time toxic matter stays in the bowel where it could be reabsorbed. There are some very good plant fibre drinks which many people prefer taking instead of eating mountains of vegetables and fruits. For more information see [Appendix K].

- **Colonics** - One major way to eliminate toxins is through the bowel. Cancer patients should keep their bowels moving regularly with bulking agents and especially with fibre. Avoid constipation. Colonic irrigations are probably the most effective way of removing garbage from the body. Correctly performed they are comfortable and leave you feeling healthier and cleansed. Enemas can also be used, though they tend to be more exhausting; they can be done at home.

- **Detox in a sauna** - Increasing the temperature of the body does not damage the body's normal healthy cells but does weaken cancer cells. Sweating and regularly wiping the skin eliminates many toxins.
  Far infra red saunas are the cheapest and the best for treating cancer. Unlike conventional saunas which heat the entire room, the far infra red models use an infra red light at the far end of the infra red spectrum. The heating is less intense and also the heat energy penetrates deeper into the tissues. [For more details on how to use saunas see Appendix D]

- **Liver cleansing**. The liver is the largest organ in the body with 1.5 litres of blood passing through it per minute. This organ has many roles:

  * It stores, produces and releases glucose as needed by the body

  * It stores many vitamins, iron and copper.

  * The liver manufactures most of the proteins and fats required by the body for energy and to build new tissues.

  * Detoxification - the liver filters toxins and dead materials from the bloodstream. It also metabolises some drugs, hormones and waste products both for the body to use and for the body to eliminate.

  Inside the liver the Kupfer cells are the 'garbage collectors'. These cells ingest dead cells, viruses and bacteria, artificial chemicals, toxins, incompletely digested proteins and cancer cells. The Kupfer cells digest and neutralise all of these.

  A healthy liver keeps the body clean, protects the immune system from overload, improves metabolism, and helps control body weight.
  Liver cleansing reduces the work load for the liver, enabling it to clear the blood more efficiently and boost immunity. There have been a number of books written on a liver cleansing diet which is also beneficial in cancer treatment. [For more information see Appendix G]

- **Removing heavy metals** - If the body has a significant load of heavy metals such as lead, aluminium, arsenic, cadmium, iron, nickel, or mercury, then it might be beneficial to remove these.
  Intravenous EDTA chelation or a combination of DMSA, Vitamin C, lipoic acid and chlorella can remove heavy metals. These heavy metals impair cell function and if there is a history of significant exposure, or a hair analysis suggests there is a high metal load, then perhaps removal should be considered.

Identify and treat other causes of toxicity

Occasionally there are other toxic processes in the body which your doctor or health professional may identify and suggest treatment for. These may include:

- Leaky gut syndrome – which allows large damaging proteins to enter the body
- Candidiasis – yeast infection (often hidden). This can weaken the immunity
- Chemical or metal toxicity – due to previous exposure, especially mercury in teeth
- Chronic infections can weaken immunity and sometimes secrete damaging toxins into the gut, sinuses, teeth, root canals, tonsils and lungs

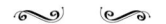

CHAPTER 3

Making The Body An Inhospitable Host For Cancer

In a number of ways cancer cells are different from normal body cells, and in most ways they are much simpler and more primitive:

- They grow faster
- They have fewer specialised enzymes
- They metabolise (convert food into energy) differently.

By understanding these differences, the cancer cells can be selectively damaged or their growth slowed, without affecting the other normal cells of the body.

Because cancer cells grow very fast, they outgrow their blood supply. Blood provides all the cells with oxygen and energy (sugars and fats), and takes away their waste. To overcome this problem, some cancer cells secrete hormones which encourage the growth of new blood vessels (this process is called angiogenesis).

Because cancer cells need to survive with a poor blood supply they have changed the way they make energy:

- They create energy without oxygen. This can only happen using sugars, not fats or proteins. They ferment the sugars, similar to fermenting a wine.
- Because sugars are the only source of energy for cancer cells they avidly take it up. Cancer cells also encourage the liver to break down proteins into sugars. This is one of the reasons why many people with advanced cancer lose so much

Cancer cells use glucose as their energy source, and prefer an acidic environment, low in oxygen

weight. [The drug Hydrazine sulphate can block this protein-to-sugar breakdown – see chapter 8].

- Fermentation works best in an acid environment, so cancer cells like the tissues to be acidic, not alkaline.

Therefore we can fight cancer by providing the opposite conditions:

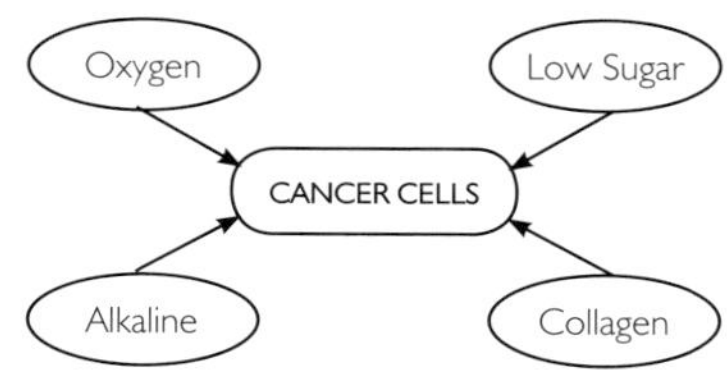

* **Plenty of oxygen,**
* **As little glucose as possible,**
* **Keep the tissues alkaline.**

1. Give the body plenty of oxygen

Cancer cells prefer to live with less oxygen. This is why a number of treatments which provide more oxygen may help cancer patients.

- **Breathing** – We all know we need to breathe to live, yet most of us do not breathe correctly – we do not fully open our lungs. Learn diaphragmatic breathing by initially keeping the chest still and breathe in by blowing out the stomach - tummy breathing. Sometimes take a double breath. Breathe in as deeply as you can and then try to take another breath on top of this. The more oxygen taken in, the better our healthy cells feel and the weaker the cancer cells become.
- **Fresh outdoor air** contains more oxygen than indoor air. Smoking is an obvious oxygen drain - both direct and second hand smoking. There are a number of specific breathing exercises and programmes which may help further. Consider walking along the beach, by a river or amongst trees.
- **Exercise** - on a bicycle or treadmill, while inhaling oxygen through a mask (EWOT – Exercise With Oxygen Therapy) this creates high levels of oxygen all over the body.
- **Hyperbaric oxygen chamber** – in a hyperbaric chamber the very high pressure forces oxygen deeper into the tissues at higher concentrations.

- **Intravenous hydrogen peroxide** (H_2O_2) *or hydrogen peroxide in enemas are treatments suggested by some. It is claimed they introduce more oxygen into the blood stream. But the amount released when 2 molecules of H_2O_2 becomes 2 molecules of water (H_2O)) and one of oxygen (O_2) is very small when compared to what is breathed in through the lungs.* ***This treatment can be risky*** *and there is little data to suggest that it increases the oxygen level or is of any benefit.*
- **Ozone therapy** - *Ozone therapy bubbles ozone (O_3) directly into the blood, or into drinking fluids or those used for enemas and colonics. Inside the body, the ozone (O_3) divides into O_2 and O' which is believed to give more oxygen. Again this is a very small amount and the value of the O' is not known. As with hydrogen peroxide this therapy needs to be approached with considerable caution.*

  Does oxygen therapy make a difference? There are no trials showing that cancer is 'cured' by oxygen therapy, but it may well help. The less aggressive treatments (improved breathing techniques and EWOT) are likely to give the greatest benefit.

2. Avoid peaks in the blood glucose

Cancer cells can only use sugar for energy. Without oxygen, they use sugars very inefficiently

With oxygen 1 mole of oxygen creates 38 moles of ATP (our energy'battery'),

Without oxygen 1 mole of glucose creates only 2 moles of ATP,

This means that the cancer cells need a lot of glucose to survive and to multiply. Make sure you understand this concept - soft drinks, sweets, cakes and biscuits are killers we do well to avoid.

Keeping the blood glucose levels low can starve the cancer cells of energy. This does not mean you shouldn't eat carbohydrates, because our healthy cells need these, especially the brain. But avoid high peaks of glucose in the blood by eating low glycaemic carbohydrates[2] It is the high peaks which make the glucose more available to the cancer cells.

3. Alkaline pH

To improve fermentation, cancer cells create an acid medium around themselves. Eating alkaline foods has been suggested as a way to neutralize this acidity and so make it less 'comfortable' for the cancer cells. Eating foods which have an alkalising action and avoiding acidic foods may be beneficial and can do no harm. Because the blood contains buffers, the blood will nearly always test at a neutral 7.4, but this does not necessarily reflect pH in the tissues. Many people suggest testing the saliva or urine as a better indication for the acid/alkaline state. [For a list of alkalinizing foods see Appendix A]. One easy way to regularly alkalinize the body is to squeeze fresh lemon juice into drinking water, eg start the day with a warm lemon drink.

4. Reducing the ability of the cancer cells to spread (metastasise)

All the body cells are held together by fibres made of collagen. For cancer to expand and spread between cells, it must break down these collagen barriers. Some cancer cells produce a number of 'digestive' enzymes to do this (collagenases and metallo-proteinases).
Some nutrients (such as l-lysine and L-proline) are powerful inhibitors of these digestive enzymes. Vitamin C is essential for the body to create collagen (in scurvy caused by lack of vitamin C, the collagen weakens and the cells fall apart). Taking high dose vitamin C can help the body to repair and replace the collagen thus strengthening the barrier, which may slow down the spread of the cancer cells.

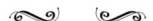

CHAPTER 4

Strengthen The Body And Its Immune Cells

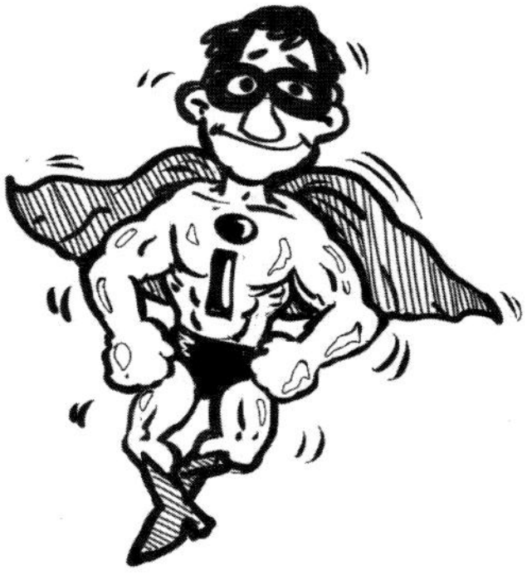

Just as a car will not work without petrol, air, water and oil, our bodies require a number of nutrients to function properly. With cancer cells 'stealing' many of the essential nutrients and polluting the body with poisons and toxins, our normal cells including our immune system need all the help they can get to fight these 'invaders'.

For people with cancer good nutrition is absolutely crucial – undernourishment can have devastating consequences as well as causing weakness and lethargy. *Almost 40%, of cancer patients die from malnutrition not from the cancer.*

Poor nutrition is caused by a number of factors:

- The cancer cells guzzle nutrients faster than other tissues,
- Some cancer cells secrete a hormone called cahexin which suppresses the appetite,
- Poor appetite and nausea can be side effects from radiotherapy and chemotherapy,
- Toxins created by cancer reduce the appetite

The answer - eat as well you can. It is often well worth having regular nutrient 'shakes' and protein powders. There are some very good nutrient drinks available which incorporate low glycaemic sugars, good fats, proteins and fibre. Such improved nutrition can make a big difference in wellbeing and long term outlook for someone with cancer.

1. Diet

An excellent diet can have 3 roles:
(1) To provide all the nutrients the body needs to function perfectly.
(2) Some foods actually damage cancer cells.
(3) A good diet can boost the immune system.

There are many foods and herbs which have been claimed to attack cancer cells or strengthen the immune system. There is much debate around these; however there is NO debate that a good healthy diet is very important.

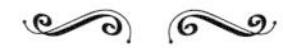

There Is No Debate That An Excellent Healthy Diet Is Very Important

- Eat plenty of many different fresh fruits and vegetables, picked only when ripe which is when all the vitamins are present. Preferably organic and free of toxins and sprays. Eat in Technicolor.
- Avoid eating too much meat or saturated fats and avoid processed foods.
- Eat saltwater fish regularly to provide good quality protein and essential fats.
- Avoid sugar and other high glycaemic carbohydrates, coffee and alcohol.
- To retain their goodness, most foods are best undercooked or eaten raw.
- Freshly prepared sprouts are full of nutrients. Many people with cancer find it easier to grow their own.
- The cruciferous vegetables are full of antioxidants, isothiocyanates and also indole-3-carbinol - which have a detrimental effect on cancer cells. A list of the cruciferous vegetables is given in [Appendix B].
- Other natural cancer fighting foods are listed in [Appendix C].

An ideal diet is almost totally vegetarian (with the addition of good fish). Using organic foods will reduce the toxic burden the immune system has to cope with. Remember many vegetables have anticancer actions, most of which we have not identified nor understood.

2. Nutritional supplements

We believe nutritional supplements are essential for everybody and even more so for those with cancer.
It does not take an Einstein to realise that many, if not most, cancer patients have difficulty in providing their cells and immune system with all the nutrients they require. This is because:

- Of the poor quality of today's food which is grown in deficient soils, picked early before the vitamins are set, and then processed.[3] All of these deplete nutrients from our food.
- Many cancer patients have poor appetites because of their illness or the drugs they take.
- The dividing cancer cells consume many of the nutrients destined for other parts of the body.
- The body uses up many nutrients as it attempts to neutralise the toxins released by cancer cells.

  Thus a person with cancer requires a much higher level of essential nutrients than someone without the disease. It is virtually impossible to achieve this with today's food, hence our very strong belief in the added value of good quality supplements which can make up the shortfall.
- Starvation of the cells is very common in people with advanced cancer, and the benefits of providing the cells of the body with an optimal supply of all the nutrients, vitamins and minerals they need seems just so obvious.

  Many medical professionals do not encourage their cancer patients to take supplements – it may be hard to understand why. It is probably because of their previous experience (or the experience of their tutors) that using the poor quality supplements of the past seemed to provide very little benefit.

  However, today there are a number of excellent supplements that are made to the same quality as pharmaceutical drugs (GMP - Good Manufacturing Practice) and that contain optimal levels of those nutrients required by normal cells to function as well as they can. (A good review and comparison of the supplements available can be found in a book by McWilliam [4])

Using such high quality pharmaceutical grade supplements can greatly help a person suffering from cancer.

A good supplement plus a good diet will provide the cells and the immune system with the nutrients they require to function optimally.

Many cancer patients take huge quantities of herbs and supplements. We do not feel that there is much benefit in going beyond an ideal level of the nutrients required to keep the cells healthy. Because the nutrients are being soaked up for the reasons described at the beginning of this chapter, possibly a higher dose than a healthy person would require may be appropriate. Note that we are talking about the optimal level of these nutrients, not just the RDA (the recommended daily allowance).The RDA is the dose required to prevent deficiency diseases (scurvy and rickets) – not the dose which makes the cells function to their perfect capacity. In the book by McWilliam[4] the ideal level of the many nutrients is discussed in a very comprehensive way.

Note - TAKING SUPPLEMENTS IS NOT AN EXCUSE FOR AN INFERIOR DIET!

Because there are many helpful and unrecognized ingredients in fruit and vegetables, we recommend people eat as well as they can and take a good supplement. Their bodies can help themselves to any nutrient required, and if there is a surfeit, with a good supplement it can be easily excreted.

We strongly recommend that everyone with any form of cancer should take a good preparation of the following supplements:

Multivitamin/multimineral tablets - A comprehensive good quality multivitamin and multimineral supplement will make sure that all the essential nutrients are ingested. This is the foundation.
A good multi tablet should contain, among many other nutrients, vitamin E, beta carotene, vitamin D (see below), folic acid, vitamin C and selenium (or this can be taken separately). There are many reasons why these are so important:

- **Vitamin E** (400 – 800iu daily) – has been shown to reduce breast cancer[5] and prostate cancer.[6]

- **Vitamin C** – Cancer patients are nearly always depleted of vitamin C, which, because it is like a sugar, is avidly taken up by cancer cells. A regular intake of vitamin C (4 - 8 grams per day) has a number of beneficial actions:
  * Most people experience a major improvement in quality of life, with an increased sense of wellbeing and improved appetite.
  * It neutralizes carcinogenic nitrites from our diet and from the air.
  * It reduces inflammation and so can help in relieving some of the inflammatory pain caused by cancer cells.
  * It boosts the immune system, helping it to attack and kill the cancer cells more effectively.
  * It may reduce the spread of cancer (metastasis). Cancer cells spread between normal cells by breaking down the fibrous collagen which holds our cells together. Vitamin C is essential to replace this collagen and so may make it harder for the cancer to spread.
  * Vitamin C given intravenously in high doses can selectively damage cancer cells and act almost like chemotherapy. [see chapter 5]

  Note - it is very important not to stop high dose vitamin C treatment suddenly because it can create a 'scurvy' like situation. If vitamin C must be stopped, gradually reduce the dose over a few days.

- **Vitamin D** – the sunshine vitamin. Vitamin D is a hormone-like vitamin and may reduce breast cancer through an anti-oestrogenic action. When the skin is exposed to sunlight it makes vitamin D. This can reduce the incidence of breast cancer by 30-40%.[7]
  Vitamin D also seems to be protective against cancer in men. Men with higher levels of vitamin D were half as likely to develop aggressive forms of prostate cancer compared with men with lower levels. [8]

  Note - in some cancers high blood calcium levels can develop. Because vitamin D can raise calcium further, before taking a supplement containing calcium or vitamin D check with your doctor that the calcium levels are satisfactory.

- **Folic acid** – low levels in the blood are associated with an increased incidence of breast, cervical, brain, lung and colon cancer. In the USA Nurses Study, colon cancer was reduced by a massive 75% in those taking multivitamins containing folic acid for longer then 15 years. [9]

- **Selenium** (dose 100-200ug daily) is essential if you live in NZ, parts of China and some areas in the United States of America. In these areas the soil is very low in this mineral.

Selenium has been shown to reduce the risk of cancer in China.[10] In a study performed in Arizona, selenium supplements halved the number of deaths from many cancers.[11]
Selenium boosts the immune system, is essential for the formation of glutathione and other very important enzymes. Selenium can also provide some protection from the dangerous heavy metals mercury, cadmium and arsenic which can be stored in the body.

- **Magnesium** - many people benefit from additional magnesium 500mg per day. It usually comes with calcium, but check first with your doctor that the cancer has not caused high calcium levels. Magnesium can help with relaxation, reduce cramps and improve sleep.

Omega 3 fish oils – 1 gram daily will provide plenty of the essential fats necessary for healthy cell and immune function. Some studies have also shown that the spread of prostate and liver cancer may be slowed with omega 3 fish oils.[12, 13] Note that fish and fish oils in most parts of the world are contaminated with mercury, so taking high doses can be a two edged sword. Fortunately, pharmaceutical grade fish oils are mercury free – another reason to use only quality supplements.

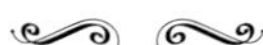

The supplements we recommend all cancer patients to take:

- ***A good quality multivitamin and multimineral – (see McWilliam [4] for a selection of the best ones).***
- ***Selenium 200ug per day – (this may be present in the multivitamin and multimineral tablet, but usually is not).***
- ***Omega 3 fish oils – 1 gram daily.***
- ***Vitamin C 4 – 6 grams daily (note that is 4,000 – 6000mg) in divided doses over the day.***

We believe that these supplements are absolutely essential

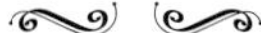

In addition to providing the body and the cells of the immune system with the 'fuel' to function as well as they can, there are a number of supplements that can be positively helpful when patients are receiving chemotherapy and radiotherapy.

- **Vitamin E**
  - ∗ Reduces lung fibrosis caused by bleomycin[14]
  - ∗ Helps to protects normal cells from damage during irradiation[15]
- **Vitamin C** reduces cardio toxicity (heart damage) which can be caused by adriomycin[16]
- **Co-enzyme Q10**
  - ∗ Helps to protect the heart cells from damage by adriomycin[17]
- Some dermatologists recommend the use of very pure preservative free 'night renewal creams' to be applied to an area which has received radiotherapy. Anecdotal reports suggest that if applied to the area (e.g. breast) after the radiotherapy dose it can soothe the skin and reduce the risk of burning. It is important that the cream contains no preservatives or metals (especially aluminium). [*For further information please contact the authors*]

3. *Juicing*

Juicing fresh fruits and vegetables has become fashionable in many areas of the world. The benefits of juicing for people with cancer seem to be well established.

In addition to the known vitamins and minerals, fruits and vegetables contain many chemicals which are beneficial in preventing and treating cancer. These plant chemicals are called phytochemicals, and many drug firms are attempting to identify the useful ones from the myriad of compounds available to make new drugs.

Fresh produce also contains enzymes which are essential catalysts, enabling many thousands of chemical reactions to occur within the body. Heating will destroy these enzymes; this is why low speed juicing is best because it preserves these beneficial chemicals. As an example, the enzyme trypsin can break down the protective protein coating which forms round malignant tissue, and may make the cancer cells more susceptible to the immune defense system. The high fibre and water content in juice helps flush out toxins. Correct juicing does seem a very sensible practice.

To get the best out of juicing it is important to use fresh and organic produce, and to use a low speed juicer because it does not reach high temperatures which could damage the contents of the resulting juice.

4. Green tea

In addition to good juice, possibly the best beverage to drink is green tea, at least 2-3 cups per day. In addition to being a refreshing and invigorating brew, green tea has many proven actions.

- It blocks enzymes called matrix metallo-proteinases created by the cancer cells to help them dissolve collagen. Blocking these enzymes may reduce the cancer cells spreading.
- It encourages natural cancer cell death (apoptosis).
- It penetrates the blood brain barrier so can help in the treatment of people with brain cancer.
- It has been shown to help in the treatment of medullo blastoma, chronic lymphatic leukemia, skin cancer, and metastatic prostate cancer.[18]
- Breast cancer patients in Japan who drank green tea had longer survival times.[19]

Herbs and supplements – is their use appropriate?

Most doctors and many health professionals have little knowledge about these compounds, and as frequently happens in medicine, lack of knowledge is often equated with lack of effect. However, there are good trials confirming their benefit, and many years of experience in complementary practices in the Orient should not be ignored without good reason. Some of these herbs and supplements are further discussed in chapter 8.

On the other hand some complementary therapies do have significant side effects and there have been a number of reports of contamination of some products with lead and other toxins. For this reason it is important that the alternative or complementary products are made to pharmaceutical standards (GMP).

Many of today's drugs are derived from plants and herbs, including some anti cancer drugs such as – Taxol (Pacific yew), Etoposide (May apple), and Vincristine and Vinblastin (periwinkle plant).

Most of these herbs and supplements are very unlikely to have any adverse effects and together with conventional treatment could be very beneficial. However if you are currently undergoing treatment (chemo or radiotherapy) it would be best to tell your doctor what supplements you are taking.

5. Other support programmes:

To strengthen the body and the immune system we need to look after our body and mind. Some ways of doing these have already been discussed in chapter 1.

- Get regular and plentiful sleep. Taking melatonin at night can frequently help. Melatonin has additional useful properties in people with cancer. [see chapter 8]
- Do regular healthy physical exercise – to a level you find comfortable.
- Engage in regular relaxation and spiritual practice (if this is appropriate).
- Have a regular massage. Consider lymphatic massage.
- Spend time with nature – woods, flowers, sea, and hills – anywhere where you can feel at peace and appreciate our world with awe.

6. New and developing treatments

These are still in the developmental phase, but some hospital units actually do provide these treatments and hopefully with time, many more will be developed. Their aim is to strengthen the immune system and direct it more strongly to fight against the cancer cells, thus enabling the body to rid itself of the cancer.

- **Peptide modulators** – These are compounds which can be inserted into the T killer cells of the immune system and could make them much more active and successful in their hunt to identify the cancer cells.

- **Cancer vaccines** – Just as vaccines help the body's immune system to recognise and then fight viruses and some bacteria, vaccines are also being developed for cancer cells. Sometimes the body does not recognise the cancer cells. Vaccines can be made from cancer cells which are removed, changed and then re-injected back into the body. In another technique, some of the patient's immune cells are removed from the body, are exposed to the cancer, and then replaced into the body. These boosted and fortified cells have a new aggression to fight the cancer cells.

- **The cancer cell 'switch'** – Many researchers believe that there is some biochemical 'switch' which makes cancer cells multiply out of control. One such 'switch' has already been found for a form of leukemia. If we can find 'switches' for other cancers, then treatment may become very simple. Many researchers the world over are hunting for the 'switch'.

The future - Over the next few years, these treatments have the potential to completely change the treatment of cancer. We anticipate that within 10 – 15 years, cancer will be feared no more than bacterial or viral infections are today. In our grandparents' day, polio, smallpox, tuberculosis and pneumonia were feared diseases, much as cancer is today. Vaccines and antibiotics have blunted the effects of these illnesses. We are confident that new treatments will relegate cancer into a 'serious disease of the past' box.

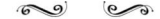

CHAPTER 5

Treatments Targeting Cancer Cells

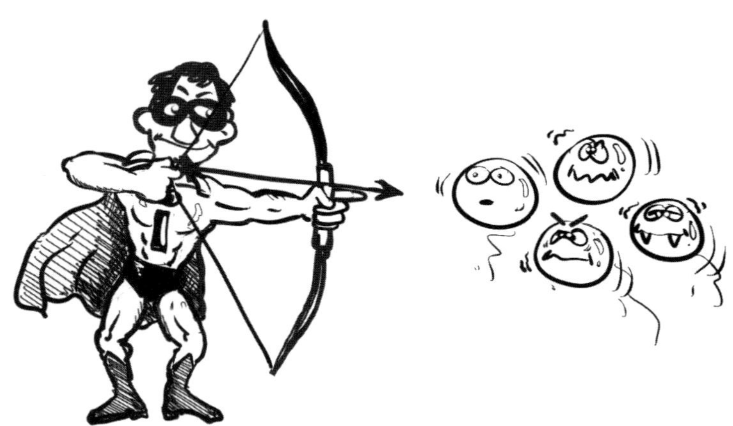

Conventional, traditional therapies

Surgery – Surgery is used in several ways to help people with cancer. It is the oldest form of cancer treatment and it provides the best chance to stop many types of cancer.

Having surgery for cancer is different for everyone and depends on the type of surgery, the type of cancer, and the patient's overall health. Surgery may be curative, especially if the cancer is localised.

Surgery can be performed to diagnose the cancer or evaluate its spread. Sometimes it is used to reduce symptoms, especially when the cancer is blocking one of the 'tubes' in the body, or pushing on vital organs.

Occasionally 'debulking' surgery is suggested. This removes much but not all of the cancer mass – and is done when removing the whole cancer is impossible or too dangerous. By reducing the size of the cancer and the number of cancer cells in the body, other treatments may then become more successful.

Surgery is often used in conjunction with radiotherapy or chemotherapy.

In some cases surgery offers the best chance of a complete cure, but if the surgery being considered is radical, then do ask for a second opinion and ask if the more extreme surgery is any more likely to be successful than a more localized procedure. This applies especially to breast cancer. In breast cancer the timing of the surgery in relation to the menstrual cycle in younger women may be important [see chapter 7].

Radiotherapy – Radiotherapy therapy uses radiation to kill cancer cells and to shrink tumours. The radiation damages the genetic material in the cells and stops them from multiplying. It also affects normal cells as they multiply. However cancer cells appear to be more sensitive to irradiation and normal cells have a greater ability to recover. Often radiation is directed at the cancer cells from a number of angles – this focuses the total dose onto the cancer cells so that the surrounding tissues are less affected. Thus the cancer cells can be destroyed but surrounding normal cells survive.

In some cases radiation is planned to be curative and destroy the total cancer load. At other times it is used to shrink the tumour and reduce the symptoms it is causing. Different cancers vary in their radio-sensitivity, and it is important that you discuss with your specialist the likelihood of benefit before considering having radiotherapy. Irradiation can be used to treat almost any form of solid tumour: brain, breast, cervix, larynx, lung, pancreas, prostate, skin, spine, stomach, uterus, and soft tissue sarcomas. It can also be very effective in treating some forms of cancer in the blood and lymphatic system.

Almost half of all cancer patients receive some type of radiation therapy.

Side effects of radiation therapy – these can be broadly split into two categories.

1. **The early or immediate effects.** These occur during or shortly after treatment, and depend on the size and area of the body being treated:

- If irradiation involves the abdomen, then some nausea may be felt a few hours after treatment. It can also affect the bowel causing diarrhoea and occasionally some bleeding.

- The skin often gets red where the radiation passes through, similar to sunburn. Do not use sun creams for this without first talking to the doctors. Avoid exposure to the sun and wash the area gently. Some very pure preservative free 'night renewal creams' can also be very soothing.
- If the ovaries or testes are irradiated, fertility will be affected. If this is important to you, discuss this with your doctor. Perhaps consider freezing some eggs prior to treatment. Of course, the womb of a pregnant woman should never be irradiated because the effects on the foetus would be disastrous.
- Radiotherapy to the mouth area often causes a sore throat and occasionally thrush infections can develop. (If white patches are present see your doctor for an antifungal mouthwash). Keep the mouth very clean, use soft tooth brushes, floss and saline mouth washes. A liquid diet may be helpful. Avoid smoking and maintain good nutrition. This will frequently mean using supplements and well balanced nutritional shakes as discussed previously.
- It is almost certain that there will be hair loss in the area being irradiated, often starting 2 -3 weeks after treatment is commenced. It is usually temporary and the hair grows back – but not always.

2. **Late side effects** develop months or even years after the conclusion of radiotherapy. These effects are caused by more permanent damage to the local tissues, and include dryness of the mouth due to irradiation of the salivary glands, thickening of the skin, damage to nerves, bowel, urinary tract, heart or lungs.

   These are all quite rare but it is important before treatment to discuss the possibility with your oncologist who will have taken these possible risks into account when deciding upon therapy. With the increased understanding of what is possible in radiotherapy, treatments have become much more sophisticated and less damaging. Side effects have also been reduced. Many horrific stories of other people's experiences are often related by friends, and cloud one's ability to maintain the positive outlook we believe is so essential. Do ask lots of questions, but be aware that this area has developed considerably.

Chemotherapy: Chemotherapy drugs interfere with the ability of cancer cells to divide and reproduce themselves. Because the drugs are carried in the blood, they can reach cancer cells all over the body, except occasionally in the brain.

Chemotherapy drugs are taken up by cancer cells as well as by all rapidly dividing cells, which includes some normal cells such as those in the lining of the mouth, the bone marrow (which makes blood cells), the hair follicles, and the digestive system. This can cause some of the side effects of chemotherapy - such as a sore mouth and throat, reduced blood cell production leading to anaemia and the inability to fight infections effectively, hair loss, nausea and diarrhoea. However remember that healthy cells can repair the damage caused by chemotherapy but often cancer cells cannot and so they eventually die. Frequently combinations of drugs with differing actions are used. This increases the effectiveness of the chemotherapy but because lower doses of each drug can now be used, side effects are lessened somewhat.

With new research, chemotherapy is becoming more cancer specific. Some drugs work by preventing the cancer cells creating their own blood vessels (angiogenesis).

Chemotherapy is usually given by intravenous infusion, but sometimes intramuscular injections or oral tablets can be used. Because of the effects of chemotherapy on normal cells, patients having chemotherapy need to be supervised and have regular blood tests. They also need to be on the look out for infections and avoid them.

Chemotherapy has the reputation of making people feel miserable. Certainly this is so with some of the more powerful drugs, and again you need to talk frankly with your oncologist to see if the discomfort is really going to be worth it. One of the major side effects of chemotherapy (and often radiotherapy as well) is nausea and vomiting. The newer anti-nausea drugs (5HT3 receptor antagonists such as ondansetron) are very effective. These drugs are quite expensive, but they can make life much more bearable. If nausea is a real problem, ask your oncologist for them.

There is also a condition now being recognised with the very descriptive name of 'chemo brain'. This condition is a combination of forgetfulness, inability to concentrate and depressive feelings. It is caused by the chemotherapy and will usually cease when the treatment stops. It is reassuring for many patients to note that these feelings are due to the drugs and are not part of their illness.

With chemotherapy, some cancers are curable and other cancers can be arrested before they progress.

Cryotherapy – This technique uses extreme cold to destroy cancer tissues. Very cold probes using liquid nitrogen or argon are placed on or within the cancer cells, destroying all the cells in the area.

Cryotherapy can be used for accessible cancers, such as those on the skin and the cervix. It has also been used in cancers of the eye, prostate and liver. The efficacy of its use in conjunction with other therapies for breast, colon and kidney cancers is still being determined.

It is sometimes used for primary localized liver tumours, and it has also been used to treat secondary tumour deposits which have spread to the liver from other organs.

How effective is cryotherapy? This depends very much on the type of tumour, its localization and also how accurately the surgeon can localize the tumour. Usually imaging such as CT or MRI scans or ultrasound is used to guide the probe, but these can only detect the larger cancer particles, not the microscopic ones, thus complete eradication may not occur. Another disadvantage is that nearby normal tissues can also be frozen and damaged.

Cryotherapy can be very expensive and in most cases is not covered by medical insurance. It is important to discuss the possible benefits and disadvantages of this form of therapy and the true likelihood of success before embarking upon it. In most cases, it is good to seek a second opinion.

Brachytherapy – This uses catheters, needles, capsules or seeds containing radioactive materials. These are implanted into the cancer mass or the organ containing the cancer. It can be used very successfully in cancers of the head and neck, prostate, cervix, ovary, breast, and cancer involving the pelvic regions.

By giving a much higher dose of irradiation directly into the cancer cells, the results are excellent, and the other tissues are affected much less. In prostate cancer, long term data show that 87% of men are free from cancer 10 years after brachytherapy.

Hormonal therapy – For some cancers, usually those affecting the reproductive organs, drugs which block oestrogen or testosterone production (or their metabolites) can retard the progression of the cancer. For men with prostate cancer, the removal of the testicles is a major decision to take, but it can make a huge difference in the disease process and may mean not having to use drugs which have significant side effects. For women with breast cancer, it is important for the cancer cells to be tested for their dependence on either oestrogen or progesterone – before any hormonal therapy is considered.

Two of the most commonly used hormonal drugs are Tamoxifen and the newer Aromatase group which block the action of oestrogen, and Herceptin which reduces its production. In the correct situation these can be lifesaving but they do have side effects.

High dose vitamin C

Although only a few units provide intravenous vitamin C therapy for cancer, we include it here because it can be a very powerful 'chemotherapy' agent, and we believe quite strongly that it will soon become a regular part of cancer treatment at all levels of the disease, and especially in the hospice situation.

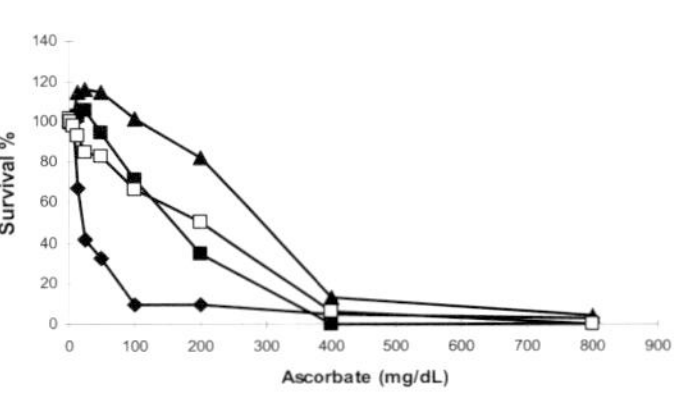

When given intravenously in very high doses, vitamin C acts like chemotherapy and can actually kill the cancer cells[20]. But the plasma levels of vitamin C must be very high. The graph shows the percent of cancer cell surviving in four different cancers as the plasma level of vitamin C rises. In these carefully performed in vitro studies, almost all cancer cells were killed when the plasma level reaches 400mg/dl. (Riordan et al[21])

Inside the body, it is only possible to reach these plasma levels with intravenous infusions.

High dose vitamin C has been shown to in some cases:

- Shrink the cancer and the metastases
- Reduce the level of the cancer markers
- Improve the quality of life and reduce pain
- Help the body's immune system to rid the body of the cancer. [22]

[***How high dose vitamin C works*** – *Vitamin C is similar in structure to sugar and the cancer cells which use sugar as their source of energy, avidly take the vitamin C into their cells. Cancer cells are not as specialised as normal cells and do not contain as many enzymes. When vitamin C enters a cell it breaks down into peroxides (like hydrogen peroxide). The enzyme catalase rapidly converts these peroxides into oxygen and water.*

But cancer cells have only 1/100th the amount of catalase found in normal cells, so by giving a very high dose of vitamin C, the cancer cell catalase can become saturated, and cannot break down the hydrogen peroxide (this is bleach which remains in the cancer cells and damages them). So the cancer cells are selectively damaged and the normal cells are not adversely affected and may indeed become healthier!

Obviously the dose must be limited to the amount of catalase present in normal cells, so it is important to measure the vitamin C levels after the infusion to determine the ideal dose for each person.]

It is important to be aware that not all doctors agree with this therapy, as most have never seen vitamin C being used in this way. However, the tide is turning and some studies in prestigious journals have confirmed that high dose vitamin C does kill cancer cells.[23]

In some situations this treatment has transformed people's lives.

With vitamin C – IT IS NEVER TOO LATE TO START, and no cancer is too advanced not to benefit.

Many oncologists do not like people taking antioxidants, especially vitamin C in high doses at the time of radiotherapy and some chemotherapy. They often ask patients to stop taking antioxidants until after the treatment. While there is some animal data suggesting that antioxidants do not adversely affect the response to chemotherapy and radiotherapy, we would probably suggest stopping them just over the treatment time and then restarting immediately after the therapy is completed.

Intravenous vitamin C is extremely safe, and can be even given in your family doctor's rooms, but again should not be used during chemotherapy or radiotherapy. See [Appendix H] for our treatment protocol for giving vitamin C.

Non-Traditional remedies

There are a myriad of additional treatments available to a person with cancer, and we have listed in chapter 8. Some, we feel, have a real part to play in both fighting cancer and improving wellbeing, while others, we believe, are of very dubious value and could possibly be dangerous. Because there are so many, we have placed them in the last section of the book. They are listed in alphabetical order to make them easier to find. Just because we list them, we are in no way endorsing all of them. Where we believe a therapy may be helpful, we will say so.

The next section includes our recommendations for treatment, and some of these non-traditional therapies will be included. Please go to chapter 8 if you would like more information.

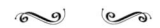

CHAPTER 6

Our Recommendations For The Treatment For All Cancers

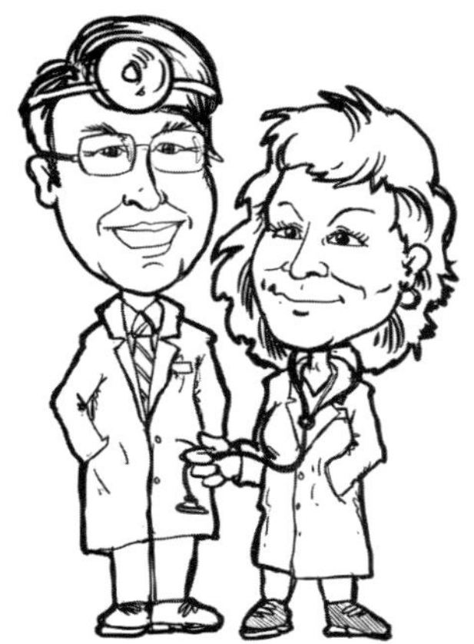

The question often directed to a doctor at a consultation is – "Doc, what would you do if you or one of your relatives had this condition?" With the large selection of possibilities available to a person with cancer, this is not an unreasonable request. To undertake all the potentially useful therapies would involve major expense and also occupy most of the patient's waking hours.

Every person and their cancer is unique, and a 'cook book' answer is not possible, and this is why we stress that this book if for information only, and not to be used as a manual for therapy. Your chosen health professional is the person whose opinion you should seek. However there are some principles and approaches which we would certainly recommend. We must stress these are only our suggestions and we most strongly recommend that you discuss these approaches with your doctor.

We most strongly recommend that you discuss these therapies with your doctor before starting them.

We believe ALL cancer patients should:

- **Remove toxins and poisons** which may interfere with the optimal functioning of the immune system, which is our most powerful weapon in the battle against cancer
  - * Eat clean, organic, food and juices, and drink plenty of pure water
  - * Dental disease – if there is dental decay, infected root canals, get this cleaned up. Chelate (remove) mercury nutritionally (glutathione, lipoic acid, n-acetyl cysteine, and vitamin C).
  - * Massage, heat therapy and far infra red saunas
  - * Bowel cleansing with enemas and colonics
- **Make it difficult for the cancer** to survive in the body.
  - * Cancer cells like an acid medium so make your body more alkaline
  - * Starve the cancer cells of glucose by eating only low glycaemic foods, good omega 3 fats and quality protein
  - * Oxygenate the body as well as possible because cancer cells do not like oxygen
  - * Go for regular walks in unpolluted areas – in the fresh air, by the sea or lake, in woods and forests
  - * Learn deep abdominal breathing and perhaps consider occasional exercycle sessions breathing oxygen through a mask.
  - * Hydrazine sulphate (see chapter 8) - if cahexia (wasting) is developing. Hydrazine can starve the cancer cells and help weight gain. (Note- read the rules for taking Hydrazine very carefully)
- **Strengthen the immune system**
  - * A positive *mental attitude*, meditation, imagery and creating a sense of peace as well as a strong determination to beat this disease which has invaded your life. Reduce stress in your life.
  - * Good *complete nutrition* – to strengthen the body, the immune system and 'starve' the cancer cells. Eat raw fruit, cruciferous vegetables, juices and limit the amount of red meat.
  - * *Nutrient-rich 'shakes'* can help by providing nutrients, energy,

fibre and protein in an easily absorbed form, for patients who often cannot eat large meals and who have no appetite.

* *Nutritional supplements* – to complement good nutrition. (Note it is important to use good quality supplements, preferably made to pharmaceutical standards, to ensure that you are getting what you think you are and to avoid potentially dangerous impurities). We recommend:
  * A good multivitamin & multimineral,
  * Selenium (200 ug/day),
  * Plenty of vitamin C (4-6 grams daily),
  * Melatonin up to 10 to 40mg at night. Note -this is much higher than the usual dose of 1 to 3 mg used for sleep,
  * Omega 3 fish oils (mercury free) 1 gram daily.
  * Only if the blood calcium level is normal – vitamin D.
  * *Other supplements and herbs* which could be added include Co-enzyme Q10, green tea, turmeric, lycopene, garlic, indole 3 carbinol, Spirulina, wheat grass and paw paw.

Two further additional approaches can help patients with cancer, and we definitely consider these for our patients:

- **Vitamin C – given as an intravenous drip** – as a form of chemotherapy (see chapter 5). It is especially valuable when conventional treatments have finished. It is advisable not to have iv vitamin C at the same time as radiotherapy or chemotherapy.
- **Acupuncture** – we have seen so many patients with a wide variety of conditions improve unbelievably with acupuncture that it would be inappropriate to deprive anyone of possible benefit from this ancient form of therapy provided it is given by a skilled practitioner.

These are our thoughts:

From our research, we believe there is sufficient data that these treatments can only be of benefit, and have little or no possibility of being harmful. Although the list may seem long, these suggestions are very easy to include in a healthy cancer recovery lifestyle.

This should be the complementary treatment approach that ALL people with cancer should take.

Thereafter it is really a matter of careful consideration exploring what therapies should be added.

We believe it is essential to retain confidence and a close working relationship with your oncologist. Be frank and ask for an open discussion about the potential benefits and problems associated with any treatment being suggested. Do take someone you trust with you and your beautiful note book so you remember salient points. Conventional therapies (chemotherapy, radiotherapy and surgery) still remain by far the most likely treatments to cure the cancer or give long term remissions.

Conventional therapies remain the treatments most likely to cure cancer or give long term remissions.

Most of these other therapies enhance this benefit and importantly, improve the quality of life.

With a combination of all of the above treatments, people with cancer and their relatives can feel confident that they have given their best shot to both defeat the cancer and have an optimal quality of life. While it may well be difficult to cure cancer, slowing the disease process down, strengthening the body and improving a sense of well being may have benefits far beyond our current hopes.

With all the research being done around the world to defeat cancer and now HIV/Aids, an enormous amount of new information is being discovered. The switch that makes the cancer cells start multiplying out of control is waiting to be discovered. The 'switch' has been found in one form of leukemia and it is likely that the 'switch' for other cancers exists and will be found. When this happens cancer will no longer be a feared disease.

So in the immortal words of an ageing Winston Churchill, giving possibly the shortest but most memorable speech of all time:

"Never, never, never – give up!"

The cure may be just around the corner, so even though treatments may not cure the disease, slowing down its progression allows scientists time to come up with the answers.

And probably equally important, many of these therapies also greatly improve the quality of life.

CHAPTER 7

Treatments For Specific Forms Of Cancer

Please do not look at this chapter as a 'cook book' for treating a particular cancer. The purpose of this book is not to tell people what to do, but to show them what therapies are available and explain how they work. With cancer, as with all serious conditions, it is important to have a specialised doctor (oncologist, surgeon, radiotherapist, physician…) conducting the therapeutic orchestra. However if the musicians know what each of them is doing and why, the resultant music will be that much sweeter. A patient who knows about all forms of treatment can make educated decisions when he or she discusses them with their 'conductor'.

The previous chapter "Our recommendations" applies to all forms of cancer.

In addition there are some therapies which apply specifically to individual cancer types. This chapter is by no means comprehensive but we felt it important to include it in this book.

Breast Cancer

Please read the notes at the top of this section (Treatment for all cancers). Do not use these notes as anything more than a guide to what therapies are available.

- **Surgery** - The amount of breast tissue which should be removed has been subject to huge discussions. This can vary from a lumpectomy right through to radical mastectomy which includes breast, underlying muscles, and lymph nodes. Discuss this carefully with your surgeon. Currently many surgeons prefer lumpectomy or simple mastectomy and removal of some of the lymph nodes in the arm pit. The decision must be individualised, but make sure you are happy with the option you are offered.

There have also been some studies which suggest that surgery done between the 3rd and 12th day of the menstrual cycle has a greater recurrence rate than surgery performed at other times[24]. However other studies have not all confirmed this. Talk this over with your surgeon and if it does not compromise your condition, it may be best to avoid surgery at this time.

- **Hormones** – these have become increasingly specialised and effective. Testing the response of the cancer cells which have been removed to various hormones is essential to see whether hormone treatment would be helpful. One of the first effective drugs was Tamoxifen (which blocks the effects of oestrogen on the cancer cells). A new group of drugs called the 'aromatase inhibitors' (Arimidex, Herceptin) is probably more effective in oestrogen dependent cancers as they selectively inhibit oestrogen production in postmenopausal women.
- **Melatonin** has been shown to have a significant beneficial effect on cancer cells, and is especially beneficial if added to chemotherapy or tamoxifen.[25] For more information read about melatonin see chapter 8.
- **Selenium** is a mineral very low in New Zealand and some areas in other countries. Low levels of selenium have been associated with an increase in many cancers. Some studies have also suggested that in doses of 200 – 400ug per day it may also have a beneficial effect in breast cancer.[26]
- **Turmeric** (or its active ingredient Curcumin) has been shown in animals to reduce the spread of breast cancer cells to the lungs. There is no evidence yet that it is effective in humans, but it is a very safe product and is used widely in Asia for its anti-inflammatory properties.
- **Lycopene** – while this is usually suggested for men with prostate cancer, lycopene has also been shown to be of benefit to in breast cancer. It acts by interfering with the ability of Insulin-like Growth Factor-1 (IGF-1) to stimulate the growth of breast cancer cells. [27]
- **Exercise** has been shown to reduce the risk of breast cancer developing. It is even more important once cancer has appeared (in 2987 nurses diagnosed with breast cancer from 1984 – 1998, those

who exercised at least 3-5 hours per week halved their risk of dying from the disease).[28]

- **Throw away your Bra** – Compression with a bra reduces the flow of lymph which drains toxins and waste products from the breast. In their 1995 book "Dressed to Kill" [29] the authors studied 4,500 women in the USA, 50% had breast cancer and 50% did not. The results are too striking to be denied:

  Breast cancer developed in:

  * 3 out of 4 who wore a bra for 24 hours per day
  * 1 out of 7 who wore their bra for more than 12 hours
  * 1 out of 152 who wore their bras for less than 12 hours

  In cultures which do not wear bras, the incidence of breast cancer in women is similar to breast cancer in men. When the Maori women started to wear bras, their breast cancer incidence became the same as European women. Therefore to minimize the risk of breast cancer, wear a bra for less than 12 hours.

  Although these data are from breast cancer prevention studies, the reduced lymph flow caused by a tight bra is probably equally significant for women with breast cancer.

Cancer of the Uterus

Please read the notes at the top of this section (Treatment for all cancers). Do not use these notes as anything more than a guide to what therapies are available

Uterine cancer is one of the most common cancers in women. The high oestrogen levels in today's world seem to be playing a significant part in the persistence of this disease. Hormone replacement with oestrogen alone, tamoxifen treatment or being overweight increases the risk of developing uterine cancer. (Oestrogen is created by fat, so overweight people have more oestrogen in their bodies).

Uterine cancers can affect the lining of the womb: (adeno carcinoma) (the gland tissue), the fibrous tissue (sarcoma) or the uterine muscle tissue (leiomyosarcoma).

- **Surgery** is nearly always the first step in treatment in order to remove all the cancer if possible, and also to enable the doctors to identify the type of cancer and to see if it is sensitive to hormonal treatment (see below).

- **Radiotherapy** – is frequently given after surgery
- **Hormone therapy** – When the tumour is removed, the pathologist checks whether it is sensitive to oestrogen or progesterone. Usually it is the latter, and if so, the progesterone therapy is frequently recommended. We prefer the bio-identical form of progesterone to the slightly changed and we believe, less effective, progestins used widely in drugs today.[30]
- **Chemotherapy** is sometimes also suggested. Discuss the possible benefits of this treatment with your doctor.

Cervical cancer

Please read the notes at the top of this section (Treatment for all cancers). Do not use these notes as anything more than a guide to what therapies are available

Cancer of the cervix is another very common cancer in women. Recent research has confirmed that a major risk factor for developing this condition is infection with the human papillo-virus, and early research has suggested that a vaccine against this virus will hugely reduce the risk of this cancer developing. (Unfortunately the vaccine is not beneficial if there has been a previous infection with the virus, and is of no value once cervical cancer has developed).

- **Surgery** – is usually the first line of treatment, and can vary in degree from cautery, laser surgery, cone biopsy (removing the mouth of the cervix) through to radical hysterectomy. Attempting to remove all the cancer has the greatest likelihood for a permanent cure.
- **Chemotherapy and radiotherapy** – are frequently also used, and there is considerable evidence that combining the two is most effective.

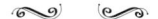

Prostate cancer

Please read the notes at the top of this section (Treatment for all cancers). Do not use these notes as anything more than a guide to what therapies are available

Prostate cancer is extremely common in older men; in fact it is unusual not to find some cancer in the prostates of old men. So although prostate cancer is common, most men die *with* their prostate cancer *not because of it.*

- **Surgery** – has become less invasive in recent years, and total prostatectomy is usually not the initial treatment of choice. Radiotherapy and cryotherapy are commonly used (see chapter 5).
- **Hormones** which lower the effects of testosterone and other male hormones (Androcur, Flutamin, Lucin, cyproterone, Zoladex), slow down the prostate cancer growth.
- Sometimes **orchidectomy** (removal of the testicles) is used. This dramatically lowers testosterone production and can be very effective in slowing the cancer activity.
- **Other drugs** which can sometimes be used include – biphosphonates (to reduce the development of osteoporosis caused by low testosterone levels), ketoconazole(to reduce the testosterone produced in the adrenal glands) and there are some data that the statin drugs (Lipitor, Simvistatin, Zocor and Mevacor) and even COX 2 inhibitors (Celebrex, Vioxx) may be beneficial.
- **Diet** does seem to be important in prostate cancer. Men eating meat 5 times a week were 2-3 times more likely to develop invasive prostate cancer than those eating meat only once a week. [31]
- **Selenium** has been conclusively shown to reduce the development of prostate cancer 10 and is also very likely to be beneficial even once the cancer is diagnosed. Dose 200 – 400ug per day.
- **Lycopene** which is found in tomatoes and pink fruit has been shown to benefit patients with prostate cancer, especially if given with other therapies. [32]
- **Melatonin** levels drop in patients with prostate cancer, and giving additional melatonin may well help slow the cancer growth. [33]

- **Saw Palmetto** is usually recommended for benign prostate enlargement, but it is also possible it may help by stimulating prostate cancer cell death (apoptosis) [34]
- **Immunotherapy** – This is a developing field, in which the cancer cells are removed from the body, changed and re-injected; or the patient's immune cells (dendritic cells) are removed, exposed to the cancer and then re-injected. (For more details see immunotherapy in the melanoma section below). Currently this treatment is undergoing early trials but it is very likely to be used in the near future.

Bowel cancer

Please read the notes at the top of this section (Treatment for all cancers). Do not use these notes as anything more than a guide to what therapies are available

- **Surgery** is obviously the most effective therapy, and if diagnosed early enough, frequently results in a complete cure.
- **Prevention** - Bowel cancer can run in families (frequently associated with small polyps found in the colon). In people with a strong family history of bowel cancer, in addition to regular check ups by barium enema or colonoscopy, we would strongly recommend plenty of fibre in the diet, a multivitamin/mineral tablet (containing folic acid), and an adequate intake of selenium (200ug per day). These have been well demonstrated to reduce the incidence of bowel cancer developing by over 50%.[35]

  While there are no data that these approaches also help people with established bowel cancer, it seems logical that if they are preventive, they should also be therapeutic – so we suggest plenty of fibre, a multivitamin/multimineral tablet and selenium (200 ug/day) and omega 3 fish oils.
- **Melatonin** – levels of this hormone are lowered in people with bowel cancer. In animal studies melatonin inhibits the growth of cancer cells and it can also stimulate cancer cell death (apoptosis).[36]
- **Cimetidine (Tagamet)** This drug is used to treat stomach ulcers but also reduces the ability of bowel cancer to spread [37, 38] Patients

with severe colon cancer with spread (Dukes C) showed a 3-fold improvement in 10 year survival when taking cimetidine (400mg twice a day)

- **Immunotherapy** – This is a rapidly developing form of therapy in which the cancer cells are removed from the body, and either changed and re-injected (like a vaccine) or the patient's immune cells are removed, exposed to the cancer and then re-injected to attack the cancer with renewed vigour. Currently for colon cancer this therapy is still in the experimental stages.

Stomach cancer

Please read the notes at the top of this section (Treatment for all cancers). Do not use these notes as anything more than a guide to what therapies are available

This is often a very difficult cancer to treat because it is commonly diagnosed late because there are few symptoms in the early stages.

- **Surgery** with removal of the cancer is the best treatment and the one most likely to be successful.
- **Radiotherapy and chemotherapy** do not seem to offer much benefit.
- **Cimetidine** (Tagamet) (400mg twice a day), a drug for treating stomach ulcers has been shown to significantly improve survival time in patients with severe stomach cancer.[39] (see also page 68)
- **Newcastle virus** – this is a chicken virus, and can be caught by humans. It causes a very mild flu-like illness. Following an infection with this virus, a number of patients with stomach cancer went into remission. There have been some trials using this therapy which have had promising results, but the numbers are very small and the benefits are still uncertain.[40]
- **Immunotherapy** – this is a rapidly developing form of therapy where the cancer cells are removed from the body, and either changed and re-injected (like a vaccine) or the patient's immune cells are removed, exposed to the cancer and then re-injected to attack the cancer. Currently for stomach cancer this is still in the experimental stages.

Lung Cancer

Please read the notes at the top of this section (Treatment for all cancers). Do not use these notes as anything more than a guide to what therapies are available.

Many cancers can spread to the lungs which can act as a sieve as the cancer cells move round the blood stream. These are called metastases, and their treatment is the same as for the original primary tumour.

Primary lung cancer is more common in people who have smoked or who have been exposed to inhaled compounds which can cause cancer (carcinogens).

- **If still smoking – STOP** – because this continues to feed the cancer with free radicals and literally hundreds of carcinogens.
- **Surgery** is the best therapy if the whole cancer can be removed.
- **Radiotherapy** is often used in addition to slow down and damage the remaining cancer cells.
- **Chemotherapy** is also frequently used.
- **Melatonin** levels are lowered in patients with lung cancer, and the addition of melatonin has been shown to increase the efficacy of treatments. [41]
- **Immunotherapy** – this is a rapidly developing form of therapy where the cancer cells are removed from the body, and either changed and re-injected (like a vaccine) or the patient's immune cells are removed, exposed to the cancer and then re-injected to attack the cancer. Currently for lung cancer this is still in the experimental stages.

Primary Liver cancer – Hepatocellular cancer –

Please read the notes at the top of this section (Treatment for all cancers). Do not use these notes as anything more than a guide to what therapies are available

Please note these notes apply to cancer originating in the liver tissue. Treatment of a cancer that has spread from another organ to the liver (from the bowel, lung, ovary and so on) is very different.

Hepatocelluar cancer is one of the most common cancers in the world.

Currently the majority of cases come from China, south East Asia and Africa, but the incidence of the disease in the USA and Australasia is rapidly increasing. This is possibly due to the increasing incidence of chronic viral hepatitis, which can cause hepatocellular cancer.

- **Surgery** to resect (remove) the liver tumour is often very successful in primary liver cancer, however it is more difficult if cirrhosis is present.
- **If surgery is not possible**, techniques to inject chemotherapy drugs, radiofrequency heating or even ethanol directly into the tumour (through the skin or via the liver arteries) may be effective as is cryotherapy.
- **Generalised chemotherapy** appears to have little to offer people with hepatocellular cancer.
- **Liver transplantation** – When performed on well selected patients, transplantation of a new liver can be extremely successful.

Melanoma

Please read the notes at the top of this section (Treatment for all cancers). Do not use these notes as anything more than a guide to what therapies are available

Melanoma is the most dangerous of the skin cancers, and early diagnosis is by far the best approach to treatment. Melanomas often look like spilled ink, as distinct from normal moles which have a clearly defined edge.

- **Complete surgical excision** is the treatment most likely to be effective.
- **Melatonin** levels are lowered in patients with melanoma, and some uncontrolled data suggest that it may reduce the spread to the brain, or shrink brain secondary deposits .[42]
- **Chemotherapy** – either total body or local exposure to the chemotherapeutic agent is sometimes used when the melanoma has metastasised.
- **Immunotherapy** – this is a rapidly developing and potentially very successful form of therapy. The cancer cells are first removed from the body. Then two types of therapy are used –
  - *Passive immunity* – dendritic immune cells are removed from the

body, activated against the melanoma cells and then re-injected into the patient. These activated cells can then attack melanoma cells anywhere in the body.

* *Active immunity* – the melanoma cells are removed from the body, changed by various treatments and then injected back into the body similar to a vaccine. The body produces an immune reaction to the 'changed cells' and the immune system then attacks all the melanoma cells in the body with renewed vigor.

Skin cancers

Squamous cell carcinoma and basal cell carcinoma

These are quite common cancers which are mainly caused by ultraviolet radiation – mostly from the sun but sun lamps and tanning booths have also been implicated. These cancers tend to remain located in the primary area, although rarely, squamous cell cancer can spread (metastasize).

- **Surgery** is usually the best therapy, with a wide excision to ensure that all of the cancer has been removed.
- **Local application** of a number of 'chemicals' is becoming increasingly popular, with many specialists evaluating whether the cancer can be removed using these before resorting to surgery – especially in places where surgery may be disfiguring or require skin grafting. These treatments may reduce the size of the lesion, making excision easier.
  * **Fluorouracil cream (Efudix)** – 5 Fluorouracil is a very powerful anticancer drug that has been used for many years. Placing it directly on a skin lesion can very effectively destroy many skin cancers.
  * **Imiquimod (Aldara)** – this cream is also applied to the skin lesion, and in many trials the cancer has improved or gone away. Just how this agent works is uncertain.
  * **Topical vitamin C** – some people place vitamin C powder (dissolved in skin cream or vitamin E) directly on the lesion and cover it with a bandage.

  Note with all of these topical therapies, the initial diagnosis must be made before treatment begins. They should not be used to treat melanoma. If, after an initial increase in redness, which commonly occurs, the skin lesion is obviously not improving or getting worse, consider the other treatment options.

- **Chemotherapy or local radiotherapy** may be considered if the lesion is too difficult to excise, has spread or topical therapy has not been effective.

Lymphoma

Please read the notes at the top of this section (Treatment for all cancers). Do not use these notes as anything more than a guide to what therapies are available

Lymphoma is a cancer which affects the immune and the lymphatic system. It is broadly divided into two categories: Hodgkin's lymphoma (which has identifiable cells in the tumour called Reed Sternberg cells) and, non-Hodgkin's lymphoma. This latter group includes small cell, follicular, mantle cell and Burkitt's lymphoma.

The treatment of lymphoma depends on many factors, the most important of which are the type of disease, its stage, its site (location), whether the lymphoma is slow or fast-growing, and the age and general health of the person with the disease. In most cases the oncologist will 'stage' the tumour with a CT or MRI scan (occasionally exploratory surgery is used) to see just what areas are affected.

It is important to NOTE that lymphomas can be very effectively treated with chemotherapy and radiotherapy, so please do not go down an alternative therapy line before giving these therapies very careful consideration. Sometimes the chemotherapy or radiotherapy can be quite arduous, but persevere, because in many cases this therapy can cure the condition.

- **Chemotherapy** – has the advantage of affecting lymph tissue all over the body.
- **Radiotherapy** – is given to the affected areas identified by the scans or surgery.
- **Surgery** – can be used to remove tumours outside the lymphatic tissues – such as stomach or thyroid.
- **Monoclonal antibodies** – laboratory made antibodies that are injected into the body to seek out and destroy the lymphoma cells.

- **Intravenous vitamin C** has been used effectively in some lymphoma patients[23], but should only be considered when chemotherapy or radiotherapy is not appropriate or has been used without effect.

Nasopharyngeal cancer

Please read the notes at the top of this section (Treatment for all cancers). Do not use these notes as anything more than a guide to what therapies are available

This cancer usually occurs in people of Chinese or Asian ancestry, especially those who have been exposed to Epstein Barr infection (glandular fever). It presents with tumours in the neck, nose or ear region causing blocked ear, nose or nose bleeds.
Early treatment has a major effect upon the response to treatment and survival, which is why we have specifically included this condition in our book. There is a cancer marker (EVP) (see Appendix J) and this together with the Epstein Barr test (EBV) is frequently performed when there is any doubt.

- **Radiotherapy** – this form of cancer is very radiosensitive, and radiotherapy is the most effective treatment. Small cancers are highly curable, and even moderately advanced lesions have a cure rate of 50 – 70%.
- **More advanced lesions** are usually treated with a combination of radiotherapy and chemotherapy.
- **Immunotherapy**[75] treating the white cells (lymphocytes) with interleukin 2 is now being suggested for advanced cases. Other researchers[76] have stimulated the immune cells to recognise portions of the EBV virus, and this has also given substantial benefit, with the advanced cancers stabilizing or regressing.
- **Some Chinese medicines** have been used to aid in the response to radiotherapy, such as the herb 'destagnation'.[77]

Other cancers

Unfortunately there are just too many cancers to include them all in a book of this size - myeloma, the leukemias, children's cancers, chorion carcinoma, sarcomas, retinoblastoma, neuroblastoma, seminoma and many more.......... For all of these, the conventional therapy of surgery, radiotherapy and chemotherapy plus our advice in Chapter 6 is about all the information we can offer at this time, but if you, our reader has any additional information which might help people with these conditions, please let us know and we will try to include this in subsequent printings.

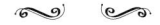

CHAPTER 8

Non-Traditional Therapies

There are many, many treatments which are offered to patients with cancer. Some make outrageous claims and create a need for dependency. Some are also very expensive, uncomfortable and not without risk. However, many may give real benefit.

We can quite confidently say that these non-traditional therapies on their own are unlikely to cure cancer, but some may be beneficial when given in addition to the treatments described above.

To make them easier to find, they will be listed alphabetically, not in the order of their efficacy. Before using any of these, we would recommend you get a reliable educated second opinion and discuss the likelihood of real benefit and also weigh up the risks:

Acupuncture - Many conventional physicians and oncologists use acupuncture in patients to help manage the pain and nausea and vomiting which can occur with some cancer therapies. Acupuncturists suggest that acupuncture can boost the immune system which is often suppressed by cancer treatments, and thus directly aid in treating the disease. The belief behind acupuncture is that in disease the body's Controlling Processes (CP) have become distorted, and that acupuncture can return the CPs to their normal healthy state. Doing this will also 'switch off' the multiplying cancer cells. However, some suggest that acupuncture incorrectly applied may well stimulate tumour growth and do more harm than good. **Therefore it is essential to see an experienced well trained practitioner.**

Studies demonstrate tumour regression in both humans and animals, but, as with most alternative cancer therapies, there are no controlled studies.

Aloe Vera juice - may be helpful in reducing cancer cell spread and may possibly cause some deterioration in cancer cells. In one trial in patients with advanced cancer, aloe vera (1 ml twice a day) plus melatonin (20 mg per day), doubled the stabilisation of the disease and doubled the 1-year survival rate when compared with melatonin alone[84].

Artemisinin - this is an extract of 'sweet wormwood' with powerful oxidant actions. It has been used to treat malaria and bacterial infections since the 1970s. This powerful oxidant action has also been used to treat cancer because cancer cells have fewer antioxidant enzymes than normal cells. There have been some individual reports of people with advanced cancer responding to artemisinin.

Because anti-oxidants may neutralise the oxidation of artemisinin, some people suggest that vitamin C should not be given with artemisinin. But because vitamin C is so valuable, others suggest that the two treatments should be given at least 6 hours apart.

Although it has been used for many years for malaria and other conditions, the use of artemisinin in cancer is still in its infancy.

Astragalus - This is a common ingredient in ancient Chinese herbal medicine. It is claimed to improve immune function by helping the white cells and T lymphocytes. Some cancers produce white blood cell suppressant products and astragalus appears to neutralise this and bring the white cells back to their full fighting function. Although most of this information is obtained from tissue cultures, there have been some positive studies with cancer patients in China, but the quality of the studies is not good enough to satisfy conventional Western doctors. However they have not attempted to repeat the work. There is also some data suggesting that astragalus may reduce the side effects of some chemotherapy. [43]

Ayurvedic medicine - Ayurvedic medicine differs from the conventional medical model which treats only that part of the body which is considered diseased. Ayurvedic medicine treats the whole person in the belief that one cannot safely split a person into parts. Ayurvedic doctors work extensively with the way the patient thinks, believing that thoughts affect the biochemistry of the body. The

Ayurvedic doctor uses many hundreds of herbs, many of which are used in a more purified form in conventional medicine. Some of these herbs (MAK 4 and MAK 5) are considered useful for cancer. Some conventional doctors have incorporated the principles of Ayurvedic medicine into their practices.

Cat's Claw - Also known as: Hawk's Claw, Life-Giving Vine of Peru, Paragyayo, Garabato, Uña de Gavilan, Samento, and Popkainangra. Cat's claw is a thick, woody vine found in the rainforests of South and Central America that has been used as a sacred plant of healing for over 2000 years by the indigenous people of the Andes. It is classified in the same horticultural family as coffee. Studies in test tubes show it improves the immune system and reduces the DNA changes which lead to cancer. There have been very few reports about the use of cat's claw in cancer but in these cases, it is impossible to tell whether the improvement was due to the Cat's Claw or to other cancer treatments the patients were receiving at the same time.

Cesium chloride - 3 to 6 grams of cesium chloride or rubidium chloride taken in 3 divided doses after meals, together with potassium chloride raise the pH, that is, neutralise the acidity produced by cancer cells. Some doctors have found it relieves the pain of cancer, and tests on mice have shown that the tumour size shrinks within 1 week. Cesium is usually a trace element, and although these doses are well below the toxic level of 135 grams, it is best to discuss with your doctor before considering this treatment.

Cimetidine - (Tagamet) is a drug usually used to treat stomach ulcers. It has also been found to help treat some cancer patients. One study showed that patients with stomach cancer lived significantly longer if they took 400mg of cimetidine[39]; similarly in patients with colorectal cancer[37,38] Cimetidine which can be purchased over the counter, was initially believed to improve immune function, but more recent data suggest it may slow or reduce cancer spread. Cimetidine inhibits the histamine production of stomach cells to reduce acid absorption, and because histamine suppresses the immune response, it was initially thought this is how it works. But other histamine blockers (ranitidine) don't have the same benefits. More recently it has been found that cimetidine blocks ELAM-1 (don't worry about what this means). ELAM-1 enables the cancer cells floating round in the blood to attach to the blood vessel wall and so become an established secondary tumour. By blocking this attachment with Cimetidine the cancer cells are eventually eliminated. This may be why this drug is so effective in metastatic tumours. There may be other actions too.

Note – Cimetidine does interact with a number of drugs (digoxin, lignocaine, warfarin, phenytoin....) so discuss with your doctor before starting this drug.

Co-enzyme Q10 - People with cancer are often very seriously deficient in this nutrient. CoQ10 is an essential co-factor in the production of energy inside the cells. CoQ10 is also a powerful antioxidant and there have been some published case studies where it has been shown to be beneficial in patients with breast[44] and prostate[45] cancer. Research at the University of Miami[46] suggested that CoQ10 causes cancer cells to self destruct (apoptosis) without any adverse effect on normal cells. Even if it had no anti-cancer activity, the use of CoQ10 to increase energy levels and feelings of wellbeing may well help people with cancer. Only the high quality soft gel form of CoQ10 is effective and the recommended dose is 150 – 200mg daily.

Coffee enemas - Enemas are one of the oldest forms of treatment still in use today – the ancient Egyptians used them in 1,500 BC. The use of colonics and enemas to detoxify has been discussed in chapter 2, but why add coffee? Some substances in coffee raise the level of an enzyme (glutathione S-transferase) which plays an important part in detoxifying the blood stream. Caffeine also dilates the bile ducts which may assist in the elimination of the cancer breakdown products excreted by the liver. (Sadly these beneficial effects are not experienced by drinking coffee!)

Cumin seeds - black cumin may be helpful in the treatment of cancer by reducing the ability of the cancer cells to produce the damaging enzyme collagenase which breaks down the connective tissue, enabling the cancer cells to spread. The volatile oils (thymoquinoline and dithymoquinone) of black cumin seeds have been demonstrated to inhibit tumour cells in laboratory experiments (including those resistant to anti-cancer drugs).

Electromagnetic and frequency vibration therapies.

These treatments have caused a great deal of discussion and controversy. While some people claim to have achieved spectacular results, others believe that the whole theory and process is complete rubbish. There are very few people sitting between these two extremes.

The basic theory is that normal cells, cancer cells, viruses and bacteria all have their own natural vibrating frequencies – much like the string on a violin, and on a larger scale a swing bridge. When soldiers march across such a bridge they are told to "break step" – not to march in step, because if they marched at the natural frequency of the bridge, it could be set into vibration and shake itself apart. A soprano singer can have the same effect and shatter a wine glass. Vibration therapies work on this principle, i.e., Sending vibrational signals into a tissue, to damage the cells vibrating at that specific frequency. The people who promote the machines believe that they know the frequency of all involved cells and so can specifically target the cancer cells, viruses or bacteria. Skeptics do not believe that such precision is possible or even that cancer cells have necessarily different frequencies from normal cells. There are a number of machines using this technology -

- **Rife machines.** The theory behind this treatment was suggested by Albert Abrams (1864-1924), an American physician who became a millionaire selling his machine. His research was refined by a Californian pathologist, Raymond Royal Rife (1888-1971) The Rife theory is that cancers are caused by viruses which Mr. Rife was able to identify using a microscope that he invented. By using the frequency of these viruses with electromagnetic fields, Rife believed the 'cancer causing microbes' would be destroyed and the cancer may resolve. He claimed to achieve significant cancer cures using his machine, but his data were stolen and destroyed before he could present it to the scientific community. His data have never been reproduced, even using the more sophisticated machines of today. However machines built along similar lines to Rife's do have some sort of bioactive effect. People who have used them in cases of serious illness do seem to have experienced improvements in their conditions. Unfortunately, the entire field is constantly brought into disrepute by unscrupulous vendors who sell machines with exaggerated and often ridiculous claims.

With the increasing acceptance of energy fields and electromagnetic vibration, many scientists and medical practitioners accept that it is possible that the 'Rife' type effect could have some benefit. However, whether the currently recommended frequencies have any beneficial effect is still far from proven, or able to be demonstated.

Energy Balancing - There are many techniques for energy balancing. Practiced for centuries in the Orient, these techniques appear mumbo jumbo to most conventional medics who have no ability to understand how it works, but as most practitioners say – it just does. It "realigns the body's energy through the chakras." Energy balancing usually involves very gentle movements of the hands touching the skin or just off the skin. There are a number of treatment schools including Reike, Healing Touch and EMF. These techniques are mainly used to create peace and relieve symptoms, so their effects on cancer are indirect. Practitioners of tai chi, yoga and chi qung also 'balance the energy flows'.

Garlic and onion - these are believed to improve immune cell function and block carcinogenic compounds entering the cells. They may also slow tumour development. They have been shown to lower the risk of stomach and colon cancer[47]. (Fresh raw crushed garlic is best).

Gerson Therapy - Max Gerson, M.D was a refugee from Nazi Germany and introduced the dietary and detoxification therapies he had developed during his time in Germany. He was persecuted for his approaches, even though his diet for cancer has an uncanny resemblance to that of the American Cancer Society.

Gerson Therapy emphasizes fresh, organically grown, raw vegetables and also fresh juices made from these. Various supplements are given, including an iodine solution, Vitamin B-12, potassium, thyroid hormone, an injectable crude liver extract, and pancreatic enzymes. The primary detoxification method is the coffee enema. Following the Gerson protocols requires an enormous effort and commitment on the part of the patient. It is said to be almost a full time job.

While the claim is that all types of cancers respond, the results have been quite variable. It is also difficult to assess the reports which state that almost 30% of the patients with 'advanced incurable cancers' have a five year survival, when the patients were also receiving other treatments as well.

Ginseng made from the root of the ginseng plant, is reputed to have a number of anti-tumour actions. There is some data suggesting that it may reduce the development of some cancers, but its use in the presence of cancer has still to be confirmed. There has however been no suggestion that it can do any harm. Ginseng is claimed to inhibit cancer spread (metastases), slow down the cancer cell growth, and increase the activity of the immune cells.

Graviola - Graviola, also known as soursop, is a small tree from the Amazon jungle and some of the Caribbean islands. While there have been many studies in test tubes showing that graviola has potent anticancer (as well as antiviral and antiparasitic) effects, there are almost no published data on its use in humans.

One slight concern is that the alkaloids from graviola can affect the dopamine producing nerve cells. Might this increase the risk of developing Parkinson's disease, we just do not know.

Homeopathy - Homeopathy rests on three principles: (1) Each substance has a unique energy. (2) This energy remains in a solution of the substance and may increase as the substance is diluted. (3) Disease can be cured by giving an extremely diluted solution of the substance which may have caused the disease. Just how this is applicable to cancer is a little difficult to understand and there is disagreement even among homeopaths as to the value of homeopathy in the treatment of cancer. Some feel it has little value, while others report results any oncologist would envy.

Hydrazine sulphate - like many cancer therapies, this compound has had a strong following from some 'alternative' cancer doctors, but was rejected by conventional medicine. However it is now undergoing phase 3 trials sponsored by the National Cancer Institute[48] and in the

USA is available to patients as a 'compassionate investigational new drug'.

Its major role with cancer is to stop and reverse the wasting (cahexia) which is common in many patients with advanced disease. The cancer cells use glucose as their only energy source, but unlike normal cells which burn glucose into water and carbon dioxide, cancer cells ferment the sugars into lactic acid. This moves to the liver where it is converted back into sugar and returned to the cancer cells. Hydrazine blocks the key enzyme in the liver needed to convert lactic acid back into sugar. Thus it starves the cancer cells and stops the body from breaking itself down to create more sugars for the cancer cells. Normal cells can use fats for energy and so are unaffected by hydrazine.

Probably the strongest proponent for Hydrazine is Dr. Gold[49] (director of the Syracuse Cancer Research Institute). He feels that all cancer patients who are showing signs of wasting should be taking this treatment, and he believes that up to 50% of them benefit, feeling much better and living longer. It can also relieve cancer pain in some patients. It has a few side effects like pins and needles in the legs, itching and insomnia. Sometimes taking vitamin B6 can help these. The side effects do go when the drug is stopped.

In patients with severe cahexia, the careful addition of hydrazine should be considered. (60mg with breakfast for 3 days, then if there are no problems, 60mg morning and evening for 3 days, then 60mg three times daily with meals. If there are symptoms, reduce to the previous dose. After 6 weeks stop for a week then repeat the whole cycle).

Some doctors believe that because of its low toxicity, hydrazine should be a treatment of choice, not a last resort. Because much of the morbidity of cancer is due to the wasting and cahexia, hydrazine, which can hugely reduce these, can reduce pain and suffering for many.

Note– hydrazine sulphate is a drug of the mono amine oxidase inhibitor group (MAOI) and some foods can react with it. So when on Hydrazine, AVOID sour cream and yoghurt, aged and fermented cheeses (most cheeses other than ricotta, cottage and cream), cured or smoked fish, meat or poultry; soy sauce, teriyaki sauce, MSG, artificial sweeteners such as Equal and Nutrasweet, , bananas, broad beans, pickles, avocados, raisins, figs, dates and dried fruit; all alcohols; chocolate, marmite, miso soup, tofu.

Hyperthermia - This is a form of treatment in which either the whole or part of the body is raised to high temperatures (up to 106 degrees Fahrenheit – some places use 113 degrees F (41 – 45°C) , from its normal of 98.4 (37° C). This makes the cancer cells more sensitive to treatments such as radiation and chemotherapy. It is usually recommended to be used at the same time as other cancer treatments.

The temperature may be raised

- locally - in a limb, or via a probe inserted into the body,
- in an area using magnets and devices which can 'shine' energy into an area (occasionally the patient's blood is heated and perfused into the affected area).
- or it can involve the whole body (using thermal chambers – much like an incubator). and possibly a sauna?

Normal tissues are usually not damaged by temperatures to this level, but the heating needs to be uniform. Total body heating can very occasionally cause adverse effects if people have heart or other vascular disorders. Patients being treated with hyperthermia do need to be carefully monitored, and their BP may well be very low when they stand up following treatment. Diarrhoea, nausea and vomiting are not uncommon with hyperthermia.

Does it work? A statement from the American National Cancer Institute shows that it is being accepted in conventional treatment regimens[50]: *"Many of these studies, but not all, have shown a significant reduction in tumour size when hyperthermia is combined with other treatments. However, not all of these studies have shown increased survival in patients receiving the combined treatments."*

There have also been a number of reports showing that hyperthermia can reduce the pain caused by cancer.

Indole-3-Carbinol - Cruciferous vegetables (such as cauliflower, broccoli, Brussels sprouts, cabbage, for more see Appendix B) have long been known to help fight and protect against cancer. They are called cruciferous because their flowers look like little crosses.

One active ingredient in these plants which causes the destruction of cancer cells is called Indole-3-Carbinol (I3C). Studies have shown that when given with tamoxifen, it is more effective than tamoxifen alone in breast cancer[51], possibly by neutralizing the action of oestrogen. It has also been shown to be helpful in late stage cancers. I3C also blocks the entry of some toxins and carcinogens (dioxin) into the cells of the body.

Most cancer specialists recommend their patients eat cruciferous vegetables, and probably adding supplemental I3C (or its derivative, DIM- Di Indole Methane) may give additional benefit and ensure an optimal intake is achieved. Some good multivitamin/mineral supplements also contain cruciferous extracts.

Laetrile - other names for laetrile are amygdaline and B17. Centuries ago our food was quite rich in laetrile which comes from the seeds of non-citrus fruits. The Hunza people, who live in near isolation in the Himalayas almost never contract cancer. Their diet is exceptionally high in laetrile from apricot seeds which they powder and grind into oils.

Cancer cells are rich in the enzyme beta-glucuronidase. This reacts with laetrile and forms the toxic material CYANIDE. Cancer cells have thousands more times the amount of beta- glucosidase than normal cells, so therefore produce huge amounts of cyanide. Normal cells also have a large amount of the enzyme rhodanese which converts the cyanide to harmless thiocyanates which are excreted in the urine. Cancer cells have very little rhodanese.

Theoretically laetrile should help most forms of cancer and anecdotal reports suggest that it can reduce pain and improve survival time quite significantly. Scientists at Sloan-Kettering Institute (one of the USA's foremost cancer hospitals), tested laetrile in mice[52] - while it did not destroy the primary tumours, some of the studies showed that laetrile can produce a 60 percent reduction in lung metastases. Following this work, laetrile is mainly used to treat metastases (spread) while other treatments are used to fight the primary cancer. In some countries (USA), the use of laetrile is illegal (this appears to be a political rather than therapeutic decision[52]).

Foods rich in laetrile include: barley, bitter almonds, chick peas, wheat grass, lentils, flaxseed, maize, millet, the seeds of apricot, apple, pineapple, cherry, nectarine, peach, plum.

Some recommend eating a few seeds of bitter almonds or apricot every hour (total 50-60 seeds) per day. If you are able to obtain laetrile tablets the dose is 500mg two to six tablets per day.

Live Cell Therapy - also called cellular therapy, cellular suspensions, glandular therapy, fresh cell therapy, siccacell therapy, embryonic cell therapy, and organotherapy. In this treatment, processed tissue from animal embryos or animal organs is injected or taken orally. Sometimes the products are made from the animal organs that correspond to the unhealthy organs of the patient. These cells are claimed to enter the diseased organs and strengthen them to fight against the cancer.

It is difficult to see how this can possibly be beneficial. When taken by mouth animal proteins are digested and broken down before being absorbed. If given by injection, the body makes antibodies against the cells and rejects them. In cancer it is difficult to see why this should be any different.

However of greater importance is that injected animal cells could introduce viral diseases (such as mad cow disease) and there is a significant risk of triggering a severe allergic or anaphylactic reaction. There are many reports round the world of severe, often fatal, reactions to this form of treatment.

Before a person embark on a series of live cell treatments, because of the risk of adverse reactions, make sure that the full resuscitation equipment is available the medical staff are skilled in its use!

Lycopene - (10 to 14 mg per day) - is found in tomatoes (tomato juice, ketchup, tomato paste and pizza sauce) and other pink fruit – melons, pink grapefruit and pink guava. This compound interferes with insulin-like growth factors (IGF) which may help cancers to grow.

Lycopene is very nontoxic but is a powerful preventive and treatment for cancer. It has been proven to reduce the risk of developing prostate, stomach, lung, pancreas, colon, rectum, oesophagus, oral cavity, breast and cervical cancers[53],. Even the USA watchdog-body, the FDA,[54] has stated that "eating tomatoes (lycopene) is linked to reduced risk of gastric, ovarian, pancreatic and prostate cancers."

Lycopene has been shown to improve the outlook in patients with proven prostate and breast cancers.

It also has anti-inflammatory actions which can reduce swelling and pain.

Anyone with a family history of breast or prostate cancer should take lycopene as a preventive. People who have prostate cancer should probably also take lycopene.

Maitake D-Fraction - an extract from the Maitake mushroom which is believed to activate the immune system to kill cancer cells without harming healthy cells. It also increases programmed cell death (apoptosis) in some cancer cells. It is claimed that when given with radiotherapy and chemotherapy that Maitake enhances the action and reduces the side effects. Shiitake mushrooms are also beneficial – see below.

Melatonin - Is a hormone produced by the pineal gland in the brain. Its primary role is in regulating sleep. When the light goes out, the pineal gland produces melatonin which induces sleep. In patients with cancer, melatonin has a number of beneficial actions:

- **It improves the appetite** – Cancer cells produce a number of materials (interleukins, tumour necrosis factor and interferon gamma) that stimulate the production of the hormone leptin which suppresses the appetite. Melatonin can interfere with these actions and improve appetite and weight gain.
- **It has antitumour actions** – It can inhibit cancer cell multiplication, metastatic spread and can increase the number of cells in apoptosis (programmed cell death). It may also help reduce the blood supply to the cancer by inhibiting a vascular growth factor that the cancer cells excrete.
- **It enhances the immune function** – It is an integral part of the immune system and stimulates both the cellular and humeral parts of the immune system.
- There may be additional benefits when given with some forms of chemotherapy.

There is some debate, but it appears that melatonin may have a real role in affecting outcomes[55]. It also has the potential to help with sleep, which is often a problem in cancer. The dose used for the cancer trials was high compared to the 1-3mg normally used.

Metformin - a drug usually used to treat diabetes that has been found to have some anticancer effects[56]. It was discovered that diabetic patients on this drug had 20% less cancer[57]. It appears to lower 'insulin like growth factor' which is a risk factor for some cancers; it also lowers the sugar supply to the cancer cells, which deprives the cancer cells of energy.

Noni - is a powerful immunomodulator and has been used to fight cancer in the islands of the South Pacific and Hawaii for centuries. It is claimed to help the body make the enzyme xeronine which "can help cure various manifestations of diseases such as cancer, senility, arthritis, high blood pressure, and low blood pressure." There is almost no useful human data, but mice given Noni survived much longer after being injected with lung cancer cells.

Noni juice tastes and smells terrible (Hawaiian Islanders say it smells like doggy-do). It must be taken on an empty stomach and often sugar is added to make it more palatable. It is believed that the digestive juices, stimulated by the sugar, destroy the Noni properties, so most of the Noni juice available is worthless. If taken with coffee, alcohol or tobacco, strange interactions can occur.

Oils

- **Fish oils** – have been shown to inhibit the development and progression of a number of types of cancer and may reduce the spread of some cancers.[12] For vegetarians, flax seed oil (well prepared) may give the same benefit.
- **Olive oil** - the squalene content of olive oil prevents some of the cellular changes associated with the development of cancer (in animals).

Papaya - may reduce the absorption of cancer-causing nitrosamines from the soil and processed foods. Like most fruits, papaya contains protective vitamin C and folic acid.

Paw Paw - not to be confused with the Papaya (which is called Paw Paw in Australasia). Paw Paw grows in the Eastern USA and is related to graviola (see above). Some believe it is a more powerful anti-cancer agent than graviola. Paw Paw affects the cell metabolism so that instead of making water (H_2O), hydrogen peroxide H_2O_2 is produced. As described in the vitamin C section (chapter 5), cancer cells do not cope well with H_2O_2 and are damaged, while normal cells with a good supply of catalase (which neutralise the H_2O_2) are unaffected.

Paw Paw also slows down production of ATP which is the energy carrier of the cell (a bit like petrol for an engine). No ATP and the cell dies. Normal cells make ATP easily, but because cancer cells create ATP by fermentation, which is much less efficient, any reduction in ATP production can starve the cancer cells of energy.

Although Paw Paw is non-toxic, because it reduces energy most in fast growing cells, it should not be given to women who are or could become pregnant. It should also probably not be used long term by people who do not have cancer, because it may affect other fast growing cells such as those lining the gut. It also should be avoided by people with Parkinson's disease. Some manufacturers suggest that antioxidants should not be used simultaneously. There is no obvious scientific reason why this should be so, and because of the huge benefit of antioxidant vitamins (especially vitamin C), we would suggest that this advice not to take with antioxidants, should NOT be followed.

Quercetin - a plant phytochemical which could help in cancer treatment in a number of ways. It stimulates the immune response, blocks the formation and action of both testosterone and oestrogens and this may be beneficial in people with breast and prostate cancer. It also appears to trigger programmed cancer cell death (apoptosis).

Selenium - This has already been discussed in chapter 4. Many studies have shown that people with low blood selenium levels or who live in areas where there is little selenium have a much higher incidence of various cancers[58]. Selenium has been shown to increase the rate of programmed cancer cell death (apoptosis) and slow down cancer cell multiplication. In women with breast cancer it reduces the development of new blood vessels necessary to support the cancer cells[59]. It may also help when given with some forms of chemotherapy.

In one of the few trials done using selenium, men with skin cancer were given 200ug of selenium or dummy selenium tablets and followed for 7 years.[11] The incidence of many cancers was halved. Because of the time taken to develop cancer, many of these people whose lives were saved by the selenium would have already had early cancer at the start of the trial. It seems logical therefore for people wanting to prevent cancer or for those already with the disease that they should take selenium 150 – 200 ug/day, especially if they live in areas where the soil levels of selenium are low (such as New Zealand and parts of China and USA). Some people believe that selenium supplementation or fortification of some foods (flour, salt) should be encouraged in low selenium areas to inhibit the development of cancer and other diseases.

Shark Cartilage - The theory behind the action of shark cartilage is that it stops angiogenesis, which is the growth of new blood vessels. Because tumours have a higher rate of metabolism than normal organs, they require more blood to get their nutrition. Shark cartilage is claimed to stop the growth of new blood vessels to the tumour, thus starving it.

There is no doubt that both shark or bovine cartilage injected into mice can inhibit the development of a new blood supply to cancer cells. But injection into humans could cause severe allergic reactions and there is no proof that the products taken orally will even get to the site of the tumour. Also many cancers do not rely on new blood vessel growth.

A large amount of cartilage is required, it smells terrible, the taste is worse and belching is inadvisable. It is also very expensive therapy.

Shiitake Mushroom- This is widely used in China and Japan and is claimed to have a powerful anticancer action. It is believed to strengthen the immune cells, shrink tumours and reduce the cancer cell spread. It has been claimed to significantly prolong the lifespan of patients with breast and other cancers.

Spirulina - Several studies show Spirulina or its extracts can prevent or inhibit cancers in humans and animals. Test tube experiments have shown that Spirulina helps repair damaged DNA. Some common forms of cancer are thought to be a result of damaged cell DNA running amok, causing uncontrolled cell growth. This may be why studies of experimental cancers in animals exposed to cigarette smoke, Spirulina appears to protect against developing cancer. Spirulina also strengthens the immune system.

Sprouts - contain very concentrated nutrition. They are designed to feed a growing plant until it puts out roots to get more nutrition. Generally, eating sprouts in the diet is beneficial, but some sprouts have additional benefits. Broccoli sprouts contain approximately 20 times higher levels of sulforaphane compared to cooked broccoli. Sulforaphane is a potent anti-cancer agent.

TENS electro medicine - (Trans-cutaneous Electric Neural Stimulation) this device is used in hospitals to relieve pain by sending gentle electric impulses from patches sitting on the skin into the nerves. These suppress pain by blocking the pain signals in the nerves before they reach the brain. People have variable responses to TENS, which is quite painless and safe. Some only have relief while the TENS current is on, while for others, the relief can last for some time. TENS is a very good therapy for people with any form of chronic pain.

Turmeric - made from the Curcumin plant root, it is recommended for all cancer patients. It has been demonstrated to –

- Inhibit cancer cell invasion and metastasis (spread) by effects on the matrix metallo-proteinase enzymes.
- Can help reduce cancer cells becoming resistant to chemotherapy[60]
- It may reduce the sensitivity of cancer cells to chemotherapy [61]
- Its anti inflammatory actions reduce some cancer pains[62].

Turmeric may reduce the spread (metastasis) of breast cancer. Researchers at the University of Texas found this compound shut down a protein which appears to encourage spread of the cancer cells to the lungs (in mice). Turmeric and curcumin are widely used for many illnesses in India and China.

Wheat Grass - is a treatment suggested by many cancer units. It is definitely an acquired taste, and is best sipped gently over time rather than the 'down the hatch' approach. It is rich in chlorophyll (which is almost identical to the haemoglobin which carries oxygen around the body)and it is rich in vitamins (over 13 vitamins, and many minerals) as well as superoxide dismutase (one of the body's strongest antioxidants). This creates peroxides in the cells which further damages cancer cells. This deep green drink is also a powerhouse of many other anticancer compounds including abscisic acid (also called dormin), over 30 other enzymes, the antioxidant enzyme cytochrome oxidase, laetrile, and many other nutrients.

PART 2

Cancer Prevention

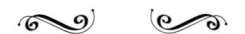

CHAPTER 9

Cancer Can Be A Preventable Disease!

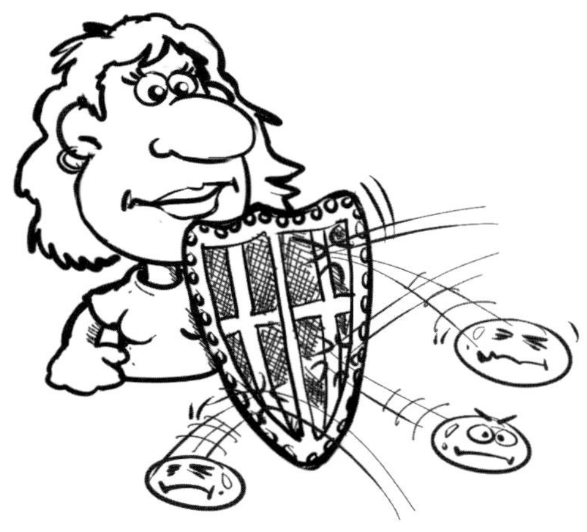

If the incidence of cancer is so high, affecting at least one in three of the population in most Western countries, it is logical for everybody to make conscious decisions about their lifestyle, diet and health which could help avoid this frightening condition.

Cancer Is A Preventable Condition

Cancer, we stress is a preventable disease and there is good scientific medical evidence to support this grandiose statement.

In today's polluted, toxic, highly stressed and under nutriented world we can no longer just hope "it won't happen to me!"

In the last 200 years we have come to believe that the medical system, aided by pharmaceutical drugs and surgery,can fix our health issues. More and more people are now recognising the shortcomings of this approach and that these measures are generally just treating symptoms - the classical ambulance at the bottom of the cliff scenario.

How much better to have an invisible friend at the top of the cliff to stop one falling in the first place!

We passionately believe that the current epidemic and huge variety of cancers could be eliminated in one generation, by those people willing to incorporate some preventive measures into their lives, especially those willing to start these measures when they are young.

This whole concept is a great illustration of the pro-active/reactive behaviour as described by Stephen Covey in his best-selling book The seven habits of highly effective people. We can choose our response. We can replace our self defeating attitudes with positive and empowering actions and behaviours.

Reactive behaviour	Proactive behaviour
If these are the odds, there is nothing much I can do.	Goodness I want to be in the healthy group!
It's in my genes, so I guess I just have to wait and see.	My genes are only one factor
I may as well continue to smoke as I have to die of something	There are many other factors which I can influence.

In this chapter we will discuss many of the features of today's world which have led to this disastrous epidemic of cancer affecting our generation. By making relatively simple changes, starting from childhood, we could be part of the movement to wipe out this modern day scourge. Although it is impossible to be 100% certain that all of these factors affect cancer, there is a great deal of suspicion about them, and making the changes suggested can only improve our general health, as well as probably reducing the risk of cancer developing at the same time.

1. *A healthy lifestyle* – How we live can affect our immune system, the production of toxic cancer-creating free radicals, and also make it easier for cancer cells to develop and slip through our body's defense systems. Many of these lifestyle changes have been recommended for years, and cannot only help reduce cancer but also many more of today's chronic diseases.

a. **Reduce stress** – Very few people in today's world do not suffer from stress and we are now appreciating how strong the mind-body relationship is in developing diseases. Stress creates free radicals; it changes our hormones, and causes other changes within our body which make it easier for cancer to develop, and, more importantly to grow.

   It is interesting that many people looking after cancer patients have noted that "cancer seems to affect the nice people". One wonders whether this may be due to the fact that nice people are better at bottling up their feelings inside. Everybody is stressed and it is much healthier to take time to deal with any stress and get rid of the feelings, rather than suppressing them.

   Take time out, eliminate anger, frustration, hatred – move towards a forgiving peaceful caring lifestyle. Don't bottle feelings up inside; they can develop into a lethal time bomb. Find an acceptable outlet for these feelings, if you have a garden, go and dig in it!

b. **Regular exercise** – Exercise has many preventative actions, including boosting the immune system, helping us to breathe more deeply thereby oxygenating the tissues and keeping us closer to our ideal weight.

   We don't have to become marathon runners to achieve these benefits. Just walk regularly in the open air, best of all among the trees or beside the beach where the oxygen level is probably higher. Exercise has been shown to lower the risk of developing colon and breast cancer.

c. **Eat as well as we can** – Although we talk below about the need for taking nutritional supplements, the benefits of eating good food have been well demonstrated the world over. One of the major differences between the cancer incidence in various countries is found in the diet of the local population. (The people in the Hunza Valley in Pakistan have virtually no cancer; they eat ground up apricot kernels on a regular basis). There are many compounds in food which we have yet to understand or identify that have major cancer preventing actions.

   It is strongly recommended that everybody should eat plenty of fruit and vegetables – as fresh as possible. Because of the presence of many sprays, toxins and other materials in our food, many people

believe that we should be moving towards organic food sources, especially fruit and vegetables which are frequently eaten raw or only lightly cooked. Eat in Technicolor; the different colours of fruits and vegetables relate to different anti-cancer compounds.
The cruciferous vegetables (see Appendix B) contain cancer preventive substances such as indol-3-carbinole – try to include them in your routine diet. Cook them in appetising ways so that young children enjoy them from the start (remember that 'mum's cooking is always best', but only when it tastes nice.)

d. **Drink tea** – In many countries the tea ceremony has major cultural significance. Although all teas do contain some anti-cancer compounds, green teas especially are a rich source of catechins which have been shown to inhibit the growth of cancer.
e. **Alcohol** – Without wanting to be killjoys, we would recommend a reasonably conservative approach to drinking alcohol. There is quite strong evidence, particularly in women with breast cancer, that a high alcohol intake (greater than two drinks per day) is associated with an increased incidence of cancer. (It is also associated with an increased incidence of heart failure, cirrhosis of the liver, family violence, and traffic accidents.). Whilst having nothing against having one or two drinks daily, any more can be positively harmful.
f. **Garlic** – There are many studies showing the cancer protective action of this herb and in those countries where garlic is used extensively, the incidence of cancer is lower. The only problem with garlic is the effect on the breath, but if everybody ate garlic, no one would notice!
g. **Meat proteins** – It is probably best not to eat too much red meat, but especially do not overcook it. Barbecues are especially bad, creating very powerful cancer-creating products (carcinogens). However, a little red meat lightly cooked, is quite healthy, but as in most eastern countries, the meat should only be a small rather than the major portion of the meal.

h. **Fish**, on the other hand, is an extremely healthy protein, containing especially the omega 3 oils which have powerful anti-cancer affects. This may also protect against heart disease. These oils are present in the fat of deep sea fish or fish which live in very cold waters –lesser amounts are found in warmer water and farmed fish. Another real problem with fish is the presence of mercury, which is both toxic and possibly carcinogenic. This mercury comes not only from toxic pollution, but because levels are high in volcanic soil, and water running off from these soils creates high levels of mercury in the sea. For this reason the United States Food and Drug Administration FDA) has recommended that pregnant women should not eat less than one fish meal per week because mercury may cause brain damage in their unborn child. The safest way to achieve the benefits of omega-3 oils without mercury toxicity is to take a good high quality fish oil or if you are vegetarian, a flax seed oil supplement (see number 5 below).

2. *Avoid products which are possibly carcinogenic*

a. **Remove toxic materials from your house.** Read labels to see which cleaning products and health care products contain harmful chemicals such as propylene glycol, sodium laurel sulphate, preservatives such as parabens, dioxins from most plastics. Look for sources of toxins within our bodies: mercury amalgams, root canals, parasites. Avoid food containing aflatoxins (bread made from old flour, bread in un-vented plastic bags, maybe packaged cereals and aged cheeses).

b. **Cosmetics** – Can contain a number of very toxic and potentially carcinogenic compounds: talcum powder is quite similar to asbestos, DEA (diethanolamine which is a wetting agent in shampoos), Lindane (hexachlorocyclohexane) is a pesticide found in lice shampoos, Black permanent hair dyes containing coal tar, Lanolin is commonly contaminated with carcinogenic DDT, artificial colours (blue 1 and green 3 have been shown to be carcinogenic), and cosmetics containing silica should be avoided . The answer – use a brand known to be toxin and preferably preservative free.

c. **Household chemicals** – Over 70,000 chemicals are in commercial production and the long term effect is only known for a minute number of them. The answer is to avoid exposure as much as possible. Don't breath in fumes, don't let them touch the skin or enter the body. Leave the chemicals in their original containers and never put into drink bottles. Never mix products unless instructed to, don't eat or drink in contaminated areas and always use in well ventilated areas. There are usually some non-toxic and much safer alternatives, and for the sake of your family it may be worth discussing this at your local health or organic store.

d. **Sprays and pesticides** – Unfortunately these have become part of modern day living, from the fly spray we use in our houses to highly toxic sprays used on our food. These can be absorbed into our body by eating and drinking, through our skin, or inhaling through our lungs. If possible it is best to avoid these as much as possible. Wear protective masks and clothing and wash thoroughly before eating and drinking after exposure. Always carefully read the label of any product you use, and it is sometimes quite alarming to see just what we are exposing our family to (read the back of your fly spray can).

3. Radiation – In today's world we are exposed to an enormous amount of radiation, and because of this it is difficult to isolate any one particular source as causing problems. So while there is little concrete data, just as with other potential cancer-creating exposures, it is much better to be safe than sorry.

a. **Solar radiation** – With the increasing hole in the ozone layer, people are becoming more concerned about the carcinogenic effect of sunlight on the skin. There is no doubt that prolonged exposure to the sun is a proven cause of many skin cancers, and should be avoided.

b. **Mobile phones** – There is a real worry about these, especially with children who use them heavily, because the radiation is so close to their brain, and their skull bones are so 'thin'. Use mobile phones for as short a time as possible, switch from ear to ear when using the phone, use air tubes to the ear piece, don't 'holster' them near the testicles or the ovaries.

c. **Magnetic fields** from power lines and our electrical systems are believed by some to sap your inmmune system, and although magnetic fields have not been proven to cause cancer, it seems prudent not to live under electric pylons or sleep with the electric blanket on (it is probably best to unplug it before you go to bed). Keep anything electrical at least a metre away from where you sleep or sit for prolonged periods of time. Consider whether you really need your microwave which certainly changes the molecular structure of foods, but may well be dangerous in its own right.

d. **Radioactive radiation** – Radon is a gas released from natural uranium in the soil, and has been shown to cause cancer in some areas where the natural level of uranium is high.

One very concerning aspect of modern warfare is the use of depleted uranium as an anti-tank weapon. Shells made from this uranium vaporize and enter the soil and dust, unfortunately remaining radioactive for many tens of thousands of years. Depleted uranium is being routinely used by Western so-called 'liberating forces' around the world. The long-term effects of this depleted uranium in the soil of those countries could be horrendous[63.] Already the incidence of cancer and birth defects has increased many fold. In our minds, we feel this use of radioactive uranium is absolutely unconscionable as is the "Aid" given to developing countries in the form of insecticides, now deemed far too toxic and banned from use in most western countries. But these topics are not within the scope of this book.

4. *Cigarette smoking and secondary smoking* (inhaling someone else's smoke) are both really no brainers. The data is so strong that cigarette smoke and its contained toxins cause cancer to develop in every organ they touch: the lips, tongue, pharynx, trachea, bronchi, lungs, oesophagus and bladder. N**othing more needs to be said.**

5. *Nutritional supplements* – While an adequate diet **should** contain all the protective nutrients, in today's world unfortunately our food quality is poor, and the level of free radicals, stress and toxins is so high that we need a superabundance of many nutrients. We adamantly believe that the only way to achieve this superabundance is to consume high quality nutritional supplements made to pharmaceutical standards, with comprehensive and guaranteed ingredients [4]. It is important that these supplements are highly bioavailable (well absorbed), enabling them to reach the body's cells. Potentially toxic contaminants can sometimes be included in supplements, thus the need for pharmaceutical grade products which are guaranteed to be pure.

The law in most countries requires only that nutritional supplements only need to conform to food standard guidelines. This is a very hit and miss standard, and is not reliable enough to tackle the need for the superabundant protective measures needed to prevent cancer. There are a few companies voluntarily manufacturing supplements to the same rigorous standards set for pharmaceutical drugs, i.e. Pharmaceutical grade. This grade of supplements has marked benefits to overall health generally- and almost certainly is essential for a protective effect.

There are very strong epidemiological data that suggest that taking supplements can indeed reduce the risk of cancer developing:

a. **Multivitamins/multiminerals (containing folic acid)** – Reduce the risk of developing colon cancer (75%), and breast cancer in women who drink alcohol (39 %).[64]

b. **Vitamin E** in elderly people reduced cancer by 59%.[65]

c. **Selenium** seems to have very powerful anticancer action, especially in countries where the natural soil level of selenium is low. In a number of studies the incidence of many cancers (prostate, colon, rectum, lung) were all reduced by 50% or more just by taking supplemental selenium 200ug per day.[10]

d. **Omega 3 fish oils** – Eating plenty of fish or fish oils can reduce prostate cancer 2 – 3 fold. [66]

6. *Hormones and cancer –*

Many doctors and health professionals working in this field believe that in today's world, women generally are hormonally imbalanced. They are exposed to too many oestrogen like materials (xeno-oestrogens) with insufficient protective progesterone.[67]

* Women who have their first baby at a younger age and those who have had several children both have a lower risk of subsequently developing breast cancer[68]. Those who breast-feed for a longer period of time also lower the risk, but to a lesser degree.
* Oral contraceptives may increase the risk of women developing breast, cervical and liver cancer, but they are protective against ovarian and endometrial cancers.

* Hormone replacement therapy (HRT), which for many years was encouraged in postmenopausal women, has been shown to increase the risk of breast cancer[69].

Breast cancer – There are a number of simple and sensible actions which can reduce the risk of developing this frightening disease. Breast fat stores many of the chemicals and toxins which enter the body. Alarming reports of large concentrations of toxic household cleaners found in women's breast milk[70] shows just how serious this is. Wearing a bra can prevent these chemicals from being flushed out of the breast via the lymph vessels. Having these toxins stagnating in breast tissue, could be a major factor in the development of breast cancer.

- **Don't wear a bra more than 12 hours per day** (This section was described in the section on breast cancer, but we feel it is so important, especially for young women, that we repeat it again in this preventive section). The 'burn the bra' movement in the 1950's might have been more a therapy than a fashion fad – had it been implemented long term. In their 1995 book "Dressed to Kill" [29] the authors investigated 4,500 women in the USA, ½ of whom had breast cancer, and the other ½ did not. The results are too striking to be ignored:

  Breast cancer developed in:
  * 3 out of 4 who wore a bra for 24 hours per day
  * 1 out of 7 who wore their bra for more than 12 hours
  * 1 out of 152 who wore their bras for less than 12 hours

  In non-bra wearing cultures, the incidence of breast cancer in women is similar to men, and when Maori women converted to bra wearing, their breast cancer incidence became the same as that of European women. So to minimize the risk of breast cancer, wear a bra for less than 12 hours daily.

- **A regular breast massage** helps the lymphatic tissue take the toxins away. Using massage oil, gently massage the breasts up and outwards -towards the shoulder and arm pit. You can either do this yourself, or, maybe much more fun - have your partner help you!

- **Pregnancy -** Women who have their babies before 25 – 30 years of age reduce the risk of subsequent breast cancer. If a person has a strong family history of breast cancer, it might be advisable to consider having children earlier in life rather than later if this is feasible and so achieve this protective effect.
- **Under-arm deodorants** – the evidence for the role of deodorants in breast canccer is still unclear. In one 2002 study there was no difference between women who shaved their armpits and used deodorants, from those who didn't. But another study suggested that women who shaved and used deodorants may have developed breast cancer at a younger age[71]. Parabens found in deodorants may act like oestrogen and perhaps increase the cancer risk. A study showed 18 out of 20 breast tumours contained the preservative parabens[72]. (However, to be fair, just because parabens is present does not necessarily prove that it caused the cancer).
- **Breast implants** – so far there is no evidence that silicone or other implants increase the risk of developing cancer, although there is some suggestion that the cancer may be more difficult to detect and diagnose.

Cervical cancer is believed to be caused by the human papilloma virus. A recent study[73] (Future II) has shown that a vaccine against this virus virtually eliminates the development of cervical cancer. Whether all women should have this vaccine or just those at risk, is still being considered. It is also of no value in women who are already infected with the virus – these women will continue to require regular PAP smears.

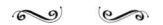

CHAPTER 10

Concluding Comments

This book has become much larger than we had initially intended. The more we looked at the problems faced by a person newly diagnosed with cancer, the more we realised that it was our duty to sift through the plethora of information and to provide a little guidance. We hope that we have been able to provide uplifting ideas and positivity in an area so often considered to be scary and final. Because it does not need to be so!

- *The plethora of therapies,* claims and counter claims must be bewildering for a person who is in a state of shock and turmoil, and less able than usual to make rational decisions. Which therapy may be a straw worth clutching?

- *We hope that you accept our suggestions that conventional therapy should be the foundation for all treatment regimes.* If the treatment is likely to be radical or debilitating, then check that it will provide the desired results. Many of the other 'complementary' treatments are also very powerful, and in the right situations can greatly increase the possibility of cure, in addition to improving the quality and length of life.

- *We all have a finite time on this planet*, for some this may be less than others, but we should strive to make that time as pleasant and fulfilling as possible. What is to be gained by increasing one's lifespan from 6 to 9 months with powerful treatments, if most of that time involves suffering and discomfort? Discuss this with your doctors before undergoing the more unpleasant forms of therapy.

- *Confidence in your clinical advisors and a positive attitude* to your health and future are possibly the most powerful medicine. We hope that increased understanding of the available treatments may help.

- *Nourish and strengthen your body* with good food (preferably organic) and quality nutritional supplements. 'Starvation' of our cells is one of the most debilitating features of cancer, weakening the immune system and sapping your energy.
- *It is important to face the spiritual side of life*, develop a sense of peace and confidence which is again very powerful 'medicine'. Remove all the hatred, anger and negative feelings of the past. Forgive those who have hurt you in the past, because the remaining resentment only hurts you. Fill your heart with peaceful, loving and positive emotions.

Talk openly with others about your feelings and concerns but, don't make cancer the only focus of conversation. Continue to build relationships with people as normally as possible. This applies particularly to visiting people who have cancer. Treat them as you would any friend., respecting their need to talk or be reassured, to discuss the future or the past. Remember to laugh and to have fun, but also sometimes to cry. One of the unexpected bonuses of cancer is that it frequently allows people time to look at the precious things of life, and many people have stated that all their senses are sharpened- colours look richer, and smells more intense. Let's take the time to listen to birdsong, and smell the roses, laugh at the antics of children and animals and wonder at the marvels of nature.

Remember that the statistics for cancer cure and survival continue to improve; it is only a matter of time before we will find the cause for this chaotic multiplication of cells that is cancer. When we fully understand the cause, then a genuine cure will just be around the corner. We are quite sure that time is not far away.

Gerald & Monica Lewis

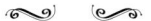

Appendix A

Alkalinising Foods

Cancer cells like to live in an acid medium. The acidity/alkalinity (pH) of the blood will usually remain at about 7.4 because of buffers in the blood. However this does not reflect the situation of the cells. You can measure the acidity/alkalinity (pH) of your body quite simply by dipping a piece of litmus paper into some saliva produced at least 2 hours after a meal. The paper should be a blue colour if alkaline and red if the saliva is acid. Pool and spa test kits can also be used. Eating alkaline forming foods makes the body less 'hospitable' for the cancer cells.

There are many foods considered to be alkaline-forming and thus helpful to people who wish to raise their pH. These include:

VEGETABLES

Garlic
Asparagus
Fermented Veggies
Watercress
Beets
Broccoli
Brussel sprouts
Cabbage
Carrot
Cauliflower
Celery
Chard
Chlorella
Collard Greens
Cucumber
Eggplant
Kale
Kohlrabi
Lettuce
Mushrooms
Mustard Greens
Dulce
Dandelions
Edible Flowers
Onions
Parsnips (high glycemic)
Peas
Peppers
Pumpkin
Rutabaga
Sea Veggies
Spirulina
Sprouts
Squashes
Alfalfa
Barley Grass
Wheat Grass
Wild Greens
Nightshade Veggies

FRUITS

Apple
Apricot
Avocado
Banana (high glycemic)
Cantaloupe
Cherries
Currants
Dates/Figs
Grapes
Grapefruit
Lime
Honeydew Melon
Nectarine
Orange
Lemon
Peach
Pear
Pineapple
All Berries
Tangerine
Tomato
Tropical Fruits
Watermelon

PROTEIN

Eggs
Whey Protein Powder
Cottage Cheese
Chicken Breast
Yogurt
Almonds
Chestnuts
Tofu (fermented)
Flax Seeds
Pumpkin Seeds
Tempeh (fermented)
Squash Seeds
Sunflower Seeds
Millet
Sprouted Seeds
Nuts

OTHER

Apple Cider Vinegar
Bee Pollen
Lecithin Granules
Probiotic Cultures
Green Juices
Veggies Juices
Fresh Fruit Juice
Organic Milk (unpasteurized)
Mineral Water
Alkaline Antioxidant Water
Green Tea
Herbal Tea
Dandelion Tea
Ginseng Tea
Banchi Tea
Kombucha

SPICES/SEASONINGS

Cinnamon
Curry
Ginger
Mustard
Chili Pepper
Sea Salt
Miso
Tamari
All Herbs

ORIENTAL VEGETABLES

Maitake
Daikon
Dandelion Root
Shitake
Kombu
Reishi
Nori
Umeboshi
Wakame
Sea Veggies

SWEETENERS

Stevia

Acid forming foods – These foods are better avoided or used in only small amounts and preferably combined with the alkaline foods.

ACIDIFYING VEGETABLES
Corn, Lentils, Olives, Winter Squash

ACIDIFYING FRUITS
Blueberries, Canned or Glazed Fruits, Cranberries, Currants, Plums,Prunes

ACIDIFYING GRAINS, GRAIN PRODUCTS
Amaranth, Barley Bran, oat Bran, wheat, Bread, Corn, Cornstarch Crackers, soda Flour, wheat Flour, white Hemp Seed, Flour, Kamut, Macaroni, Noodles, Oatmeal, Oats (rolled), Quinoa, Rice (all), Rice Cakes, Rye, Spaghetti, Spelt, Wheat Germ, Wheat,

ACIDIFYING BEANS & LEGUMES
Almond Milk, Black Beans, Chick Peas, Green Peas, Kidney Beans, Lentils, Pinto Beans, Red Beans, Rice Milk, Soy Beans, Soy Milk ,White Beans

ACIDIFYING DAIRY
Butter, Cheese,, Processed Ice Cream, Ice Milk

ACIDIFYING NUTS & BUTTERS
Cashews, Legumes, Peanut Butter, Peanuts, Pecans, Tahini, Walnuts

ACIDIFYING ANIMAL PROTEIN
Meats: Bacon, Beef, Corned Beef, Organ Meats, Veal, Venison, Pork, Turkey, Rabbit, Sausage and lamb
Fish: Haddock Lobster, Mussels Oysters, Pike, Salmon, Sardines, Scallops, other Shellfish Shrimp and Tuna

ACIDIFYING FATS & OILS
Avocado Oil, Butter, Canola Oil, Corn Oil, Flax Oil, Hemp Seed Oil, Lard, Olive Oil, Safflower Oil,
Sesame Oil, Sunflower Oil.

ACIDIFYING SWEETENERS
Carob, Corn Syrup, All Sugars

ACIDIFYING ALCOHOL
Beer, Hard Liquor, Spirits, Wine

ACIDIFYING OTHER FOODS
Catsup or Ketchup, Cocoa, Coffee, Mustard, Pepper, Soft Drinks, Vinegar,

ACIDIFYING DRUGS & CHEMICALS
Aspirin, Chemicals, Drugs, Medicinal Drugs, Psychedelic drugs, Herbicides, Pesticides,Tobacco,

ACIDIFYING JUNK FOOD
Beer: pH 2.5, Coca-Cola: pH 2, Coffee: pH 4.

Appendix B

Cruciferous vegetables – vegetables whose flowers form a tiny cross. These vegetables have been shown to have active anticancer actions

- Arugula
- Beet greens
- Bok choy
- Broccoli
- Brussels sprouts
- Cabbage
- Cauliflower
- Chinese cabbage
- Collard greens
- Daikon
- Watercress
- Horseradish
- Swiss chard
- Kale
- Kohlrabi
- Mustard greens
- Radishes
- Rutabaga
- Turnips
- Watercress

Appendix C

Foods with cancer fighting properties:

tea (green & black), ginger, garlic, broccoli, onions, carrots, soybeans, tomatoes, papaya, avocado, bhindi (okra),

citrus fruits - oranges & grapefruit and lime,
green vegetables – spinach, lettuce, broccoli, French beans, green fenugreek,
mustard leaves – the darker the green, the greater the benefit.

Appendix D

How to use a sauna.

Saunas provide a number of benefits to patients with cancer.

Both tumour cells and viruses tolerate heat poorly. This is why we develop a temperature when we become infected. Saunas enhance the circulation and this can oxygenate the tissues and wash out acids. They open the nasal passages and assist the sinuses to drain, and by stimulating sweating, the body is able to excrete toxins out through the skin.

Conventional saunas consist of preheating a small room, generating quite intense heat which for many people is intolerable. This is particularly so in patients weakened by cancer.

Far infrared saunas use infrared light, and only heat the tissues they focus on. This is a lot more comfortable, and it is possible to construct one of these saunas quite cheaply using infrared bulbs in a small room such as a bathroom or closet. Note that infrared saunas do not work through clothing. The price is coming down these days making small home units very affordable. It is not just for cancer treatments - the authors find that their cat enjoys the experience! We do not recommend this, however.

Saunas are safe for most people, but people with chronic conditions may be safer to have a companion with them. Remain in the sauna for no more than 30 minutes initially and slowly increase the temperature. For most people, use the sauna once a day. (For those who are weaker, once or twice a week may be as much as they can tolerate).

Drink two glasses of mineralised water before entering the sauna, and use a small towel to wipe off the sweat as it develops. Slowly move around so that all areas of the body are exposed to the infrared energy. For men it is best not to directly expose the testicles to infrared rays.

When finished take a shower with warm and then cooler water. Avoid hot water, and do not use soap as this leaves a film and can clog the pores. Wash off the sweat with a brush or loofah, and brush all over from the feet upwards, then from the hands and on up the body. Gently include the face, and hair. Brushing may be painful at first, but it does enhance the cleansing effect, removes dead skin cells and soon it feels wonderful.

After the sauna drink a glass of water, and sit or lie down and relax for at least 10 minutes.

While in the sauna do not work or talk, but use this time to relax, reviewing your day or meditating.

Appendix E

How we can create endorphins

These healthy 'morphine like' chemicals make us feel brighter, better, happier and can relieve pain. There is no limit to the amount you can make: the more you make, the better you feel! This is why so many athletes prefer to exercise daily rather than the recommended 4 to 5 times weekly.

- Go for regular walks in inspiring places
- Write a long letter to somebody you care about
- Turn up a favourite song and sing-along loudly
- Go to a really funny movie and laugh heartily
- Lie in bed and listen to the rain falling
- Go to the beach and dig your toes deep into the sand
- Kick up the autumn leaves and splash in the puddles!
- Pour yourself a hot cup of tea and savour it in silence
- Take a bubble bath, with candles
- Get really wet in the rain
- Visit a pet shop and cuddle the new puppies and kittens
- Explore the wonderful flowers in the florist and take some home
- Watch the sunset or if you're brave watch the sunrise
- Lie outside on a clear night and watch the stars- maybe in a spa
- Buy an all-day pass to a fun park and ride all the rides

Appendix F

Meditation

Meditation is a very powerful and helpful part of healing. It is impossible to cover this field in a few lines and we would strongly encourage all patients with cancer to look at this therapy. Read one of the many good books [74]

Helpful meditation passes through a number of stages – physical relaxation; patchy concentration (as the mind wanders onto other things before coming back to tranquility); deeper relaxation (as the mind slowly clears and thoughts stop moving around); contemplation (when the mind by itself brings in a single thought and it is perceived in a different realm); then unification and illumination (deep trance like states with heightened awareness and a direct perception of new knowledge).

Regular meditation can provide, no matter what the situation, a deep sense of peace, hope, love and fulfillment not possible in any other way. Deep contemplative prayer is a very similar process.

Appendix G

Liver Cleansing

This is a process mainly foreign to Western medicine, but in the Orient, the importance of supporting the liver is considered one of the most important factors for supporting good health.

The liver essentially filters the blood, detoxifies poisons and creates sugars, proteins and fats to feed the rest of the body. It can only do this with the correct nutrition. In cancer where excess toxin production and 'starvation' are common, taking the ancient steps to support the liver can only be beneficial.

- Drink at least eight to 12 glasses of filtered water daily
- Avoid consuming large quantities of sugar and especially refined sugar
- Avoid foods to which you may be allergic, ones which in the past have upset you
- Avoid eating bacteria and viruses in food. Eat foods which are fresh,

avoid reheating food, avoid take-aways and always wash your hands before eating. When overseas avoid unpeeled fruits and vegetables, raw foods and shellfish.

- Eat organic food if possible so as to reduce the load of pesticides.
- Avoid constipation by eating raw fruit, vegetables and fibre, and drinking plenty of water.
- Avoid saturated and trans fats and margerine. Replace with Omega 3 fats.

Some herbs are also believed to help the liver to function more efficiently–

- Taurine. This is an essential amino acid required by the liver to remove toxic chemicals and create bile.
- Dandelion. The bitter flavour in dandelions stimulate the digestive glands, and in the liver activate the flow of bile.
- St Mary's Thistle. A liver tonic known for centuries. This has been shown to protect the liver from toxic damage, and it also seems to improve the action of Cytochrome p450 which is one of the major detoxification enzymes within the liver.
- Globe artichoke. This contains a bitter tonic with protective and liver restorative actions.
- Soluble fibre. This can attach to the toxins released in the bile, and prevent them from being reabsorbed lower in the intestines.

Appendix H

The technique for giving IV vitamin C

This treatment can be given safely by any general practitioner, and they may wish to know the technique. This is based upon the advice of the late Dr Hugh Riordan, perhaps the world authority of the use of this vitamin in cancer.[21]

The vitamin is given by intravenous drip (adding Vitamin C to 250 mls of sterile water) over 60 minutes, once or twice weekly:

- Week 1 - 15 grams, 2 per week,
- Week 2 - 30 grams, 2 per week
- Week 3 - 50 grams (+ 10 mls calcium gluconate) - 2 infusions per week

Thereafter the optimal dose calculated by measuring the plasma vitamin C levels at the end of each infusion, is given once or twice weekly for some months.

Aim for a plasma level of 300 – 400 mg/dl.

However by adding oral alpha lipoic acid (300mg morning and night on the day of the infusion) this enables lower plasma vitamin C levels in the range of 250 – 300mg to be just as effective.

Precautions

Although serious side effects from iv vitamin C are rare it is important to note some facts:

- There have been one or two cases reported where high dose vitamin C caused the cancer cells to die and then bleed. (This can happen of course with any treatment which damages cancer cells, including chemotherapy and radiation). For this reason it is best to slowly work up the dose of vitamin C as detailed above, especially in people with brain cancer.
- A very rare condition G6PD deficiency (glucose 6 phosphatase deficiency) can cause the blood to haemolyse with high doses of vitamin C. So test for this enzyme before starting high dose vitamin C.
- Because Vitamin C is a chelating agent, it can increase the excretion of calcium in the urine. Higher doses are usually given with 10 mls of calcium, but if the infusion makes the patient shaky, give 10 mls of calcium gluconate at 1cc per minute.
- Because most units cannot measure the vitamin C levels in the blood, 50grams should probably be highest dose for most patients.

  For further information contact the authors at CAM Ltd, 3rd Floor, 110 Remuera Rd, Remuera, Auckland, NZ

  (http://www.camltd.com)

Appendix I

Sexuality after cancer treatment

Although sex is often the last thing on a person's mind as they undergo cancer treatment, it is a very important part of a healthy life and is often an issue people have difficulty discussing.

- An intimate relationship with one's partner makes one feel loved and appreciated, and shows a degree of support often impossible to demonstrate in any other way.
- Operations, radiotherapy and chemotherapy can all cause physical changes within the body which can impact on the ability to have sexual relations.
- The emotional effects of having cancer can change one's body image and affect a person's attitude to sex and intimacy.
- Some pelvic operations or radiotherapy can result in a loss of desire for sex, difficulty reaching a climax, pain during intercourse, reduced size of the vagina and vaginal dryness.
- Chemotherapy can cause a loss of libido – often aggravated by nausea, hair loss, weight gain or weight loss which may make one feel less attractive. While these will usually subside after treatment, it may take some time to rebuild self confidence.
- Many treatments which affect the ovaries or testes (radiotherapy, surgery, chemotherapy, hormonal therapy) reduce the sex hormone production which also affects libido and sexual function.

What can be done to help?

- Talk to your health professional about any problems you may be having. Don't feel embarrassed – this is a very important part of life. Sometimes it is easier to put questions into writing, and even talk to the nurse if you feel uneasy with the doctor.

- Talk to your partner and discuss your feelings and any discomfort you are having. Using lubricants or changing positions and varying the degree of penetration can often avoid the pain which may have previously been present. Open caring talk can bring a return to a very fulfilling sex life.
- Loving, caring and intimacy does not have to involve intercourse. Talking, kissing, cuddling and caressing – just being together for each other can be rewarding and is important. Such intimacy helps both partners feel loved, needed, cared for and close to each other, and also reduces the need for full intercourse if it is still uncomfortable. It may seem strange for older people to cuddle in a hospital ward – but do it to show to each other just how important your relationship is and how much you love them.
- Sometimes hormonal creams can help improve libido, but be very careful that they will not aggravate the underlying cancer, especially if it is in the breast or womb. Discuss this with your doctor.

  Those people who ignore this most personal part of life, miss an enormously satisfying opportunity.

Appendix J

Predicting cancer and cancer markers

Scientists are gradually developing markers to identify various cancers and genetic tests to detect those at higher risk.
The Cancer Genetic Markers of Susceptibility (CGEMS) is a $US14million study that is looking for more cancer markers and how to use them.
Family History – Having a strong family history of cancer or positive markers does not necessarily mean that a person will develop cancer, however it does give these people the opportunity to regularly check for early disease which is then much more likely to be curable, and to put preventative measures into place.

- Thus regular manual self examinations, mammograms and possibly MRI scans of the breast are recommended in some centres. Some units prefer to use the newer technology of thermography to look for hotspots before proceeding with the above procedures.

- For men with a family history of prostate cancer, regular rectal and PSA examinations are available
- Because colon cancer has a higher incidence in some families, regular colonoscopy with the removal of polyps which may develop into cancer in the future is highly recommended.

  NOTE – for the reasons discussed in Chapter 9, everybody with these markers or with a family history of cancer, or those at high risk such as smokers and workers exposed to known carcinogens, should all be following a high-quality nutritional supplement regime.

Cancer Marker Tests - these tests measure substances produced by cancer cells which are released into the blood or urine. Some tests are used for early diagnosis and can track the activity or size of the cancer during therapy. Note sometimes these tests can be raised in a number of other conditions and are not always specific for cancer. We put this information [in brackets]

- **AFP - Alpha fetoprotein** levels are often elevated in hepatocellular liver cancers and occasionally in some testicular and gastrointestinal cancers. [note the level can also rise during normal pregnancy].
- **AMACR** (x-methylacyl-CoA racemase) is found only in people with prostate cancer and may help with early identification. Its role is still uncertain.
- **BRCA1 and BRCA2 (breast cancer 1 and 2).** About 5-10% of cancers are hereditary, and the presence of the genes called BRCA 1 or 2, means those women are at higher risk of developing breast or ovarian cancer. However the disease does not occur in every woman with these markers and hereditary cancer can also develop without these markers. So the role of these markers is still uncertain.
- **BTA and NMP22** – two developing urine tests to identify bladder cancer.
- **CA 15.3** values are often elevated in people with breast cancer. [note this can also be raised in people with cirrhosis and benign non malignant diseases of ovaries and breast]

- **CA 19.9** - for gastric, pancreatic or stomach cancer.
- **CA125 or CA125/CA125-II** These markers are often raised in women with cancers of the reproductive system including the uterus, fallopian tubes and ovaries, as well as pancreas, lungs, breast and colon. [note these can also be raised during menstruation or pregnancy, in people with ovarian cysts, pericarditis, hepatitis, cirrhosis of the liver, peritonitis, and even in 1-2% of healthy individuals.]

  Because these markers can be raised in many conditions, their use in cancer is confined to monitoring tumour activity.
- **CA 72-4** – is slightly elevated in most cancers, but can be markedly raised in gastric cancer.
- **CA 27-29** – is raised in 80% of women with breast cancer. It may also be increased in cancers of the colon, stomach, kidney, lung, ovary, pancreas, uterus, and liver. [Note – it can also be elevated in the first trimester pregnancy, endometriosis, ovarian cysts, non-cancerous breast disease, kidney disease, and liver disease.]
- **CEA** - Carcinoembryonic antigen is a cancer marker used to screen for colorectal cancer. [Note it can also occur with other malignant and non malignant conditions]. It can be used to identify people who have persistent diarrhoea, constipation or bleeding from the bowel to see if further investigations are necessary.
- **DR-70** is a blood test that screens for 13 different cancers at the same time - lung, colon, breast, stomach, liver, rectum, ovary, cervix, esophagus, thyroid, and pancreas, trophoblastic and malignant lymphoma.
- **EVP** – A cancer marker to screen for nasopharyngeal cancer which is quite common in Asian people. Epstein Barr virus (EBV) seems to be related to this cancer, and people with this cancer have higher EBV titres.
- **PSA** - Prostate Specific Antigen - is a substance made only by the prostate which may help detect prostate cancer early. [Note a high PSA does not necessarily mean cancer - an enlarged prostate, mechanical pressure on the prostate (such as having a rectal exam), or inflammation of the prostate (prostatitis) can also elevate the level]. For this reason a PSA alone is rarely used to make the diagnosis – PSA

plus rectal exam, DR-70 and ultrasound probably provide the best diagnostic approach.

- **SCC Antigen** – (Squamous cell carcinoma) - is a marker for squamous cell cancers, which can occur in the cervix, head and neck, lung and skin.

Appendix K

Soluble and insoluble fibre

Fibre (spelt fiber in the USA) is an essential component of our diet – to keep the bowels moving. It comes from plant cells and is mostly composed of undigestible complex carbohydrates. They provide most of the bulk which makes up the bowel motions (faeces) – there are 2 forms of fibre – soluble and insoluble:

- **Soluble Fibre** can absorb toxins, poisons and other undesirables in the bowel and cling onto them until they pass into the toilet. Many toxins are excreted by the liver through the bile, only to be re-absorbed again lower down in the small or large intestines. For this reason, it is important for people with cancer who can have a high load of toxins, to take sufficient soluble fibre. This usually means eating plenty of fruit and vegetables, but sometimes this is difficult and a good alternative is a well prepared fibre drink. Some commercial ones are available.
- **Insoluble fibre** is just roughage. It does not absorb any food or toxins, nor is it digested into the body. It just ploughs on through the bowel, keeping the motions moving until they are finally excreted. This is an essential action as well, as toxins sitting on the bowel walls can damage the bowel cells and are believed to be a cause of cancer. Keeping the motions in motion, lessens this risk.

  A diet high in soluble and insoluble fibre is essential for good health and may also reduce the risk of developing cancer. For those people with cancer, these benefits continue plus it also helps in the removal of toxins and improves wellbeing.

REFERENCES

1. More than ½ of cancer patients …live for more than 20 years - Brenner. H; Lancet 12 Oct 2002 pg 1131-5
2. Low glycaemic foods – there are many lists to be found on the www: http://www.southbeach-diet-plan.com/glycemicfoodchart.htm or http://www.mendosa.com/gilists.htm or http://www.diabetesnet.com/diabetes_food_diet/glycemic_index.php
3. The reduction in our food quality between 1950 and 1999 - Davis DR, Epp MD, Riordan HD;. J Am Coll Nutr. 2004 Dec;23(6):669-82.)
4. Comparative guide to Nutritional Supplements. McWilliam L: Northern Dimensions publishing
5. Vitamin E reduces the risk of developing breast cancer – USA nurses study of 88,000 women - Zhong S., et al. ; J. Natl. Cancer Inst. 91 (1999) 547-556.
6. Vitamin E reduces the risk of prostate cancer by almost 50%; the Finnish study of 30,000 men - Journal of the National Cancer Institute March 2, 2005;97(5):396-399
7. Vitamin D and lower levels of breast cancer in premenopausal women – nurses study 88,000 women; - Shin MH, Holmes MD, Hankinson SE, Wu K, Colditz GA, Willett WC. J Natl Cancer Inst. 2002;94(17):1301-1311.
8. Vitamin D protective against aggressive prostate cancer; - 2005 Multidisciplinary Prostate Cancer Symposium, Orlando, Fla., Feb. 17-19, 2005.
9. Long term multivitamin use substantially reduces colon cancer – USA Nurses study - Ann Intern Med. 1998 Oct 1;129(7):517-24
10. Liver cancer reduced by 50% by oral selenium in people at risk in China - Yun-Yu C. Selenium in Biology and Medicine, Van Nostrand Reinhold Co., NY 1987
11. Selenium reduces the incidence of cancer by 50% and more, Arizona study, 1700 men – Clark L.C et al; JAMA. 1996 Dec 25;276(24):1957-63
12. Fish oils slow the spread of cancers - In Vivo 8: 371-74, 1994
13. Fish oils can prolong survival among individuals who have developed cancer - Cancer 82: 395-402, 1998
14. Vitamin E protects against bleomycin lung fibrosis in mice - J Basic Clin Physiol Pharmacol. 1993 Jul-Sep;4(3):249-69

REFERENCES

15. Vitamin E improved brain function 29 people suffering from impaired mental function following radiotherapy for throat cancer - Cancer (2004;100:398–404)
16. Vitamin C protects the heart of mice and guinea pigs from damage caused by adriomycin - Fujita K, Shinpo K, Yamada K, et al.. Cancer Res 1982;42:309–16
17. Coenzyme Q10 may protect the heart from the cardiotoxic effects of adriomycin - Judy WV, Hall JH, Dugan W, et al. Biomed Clin Aspects Coenzyme Q. 1984;4:231-241.
18. The protective actions and compounds found in green tea - Kaegi E,. Canadian Medical Association 1998;158:1033-1035.
19. Green tea improves prognosis in women with breast cancer – Nakachi K et al - Jpn J Cancer Res. 1998 Mar;89(3):254-61
20. High dose vitamin C is selectively toxic to cancer cells - September 12, 2005; Proceedings of the National Academy of Sciences refs
21. Intravenous ascorbate as a chemotherapeutic and biologic response agent – an excellent review of the work by Riordan including his techniques for infusing the vitamin - http://brightspot.org/cresearch/intravenousc2.shtml
22. Vitamin C and the immune system - Vitamin C and Infectious Diseases," Hemila, Harri, in Vitamin C in Health and Disease, Packer, Lester and Fuchs, Jurgen (eds.), 1997;Chapter 27:471-503. 27873
23. High dose Vitamin C as a cancer therapy 3 cases - Padayatty SJ, Riordan HD, et al; CMAJ 2006;174(7):937-42; and Clinical and experimental experiences with Intravenous Vitamin C – Riordan et al – J Orthomol Med; 15, 4. 2000. 201-213
24. Cancer surgery between the 3rd & 12th day of the menstrual cycle has a higher risk of recurrence Cooper LS, et al- Atkins Breast Unit, Guy's Hospital, London, United Kingdom. Cancer. 1999;860:2053-2058.
25. The benefits of taking melatonin with Tamoxifen - Lissoni, P., et al.. British Journal of Cancer. 71(4):854-856; 1995.
26. The beneficial effects of selenium on the growth of breast cancer - Redman, C., et al. Cancer Letters. 125(1-2):103-110, 1998.
27. The effects of Lycopene on breast cancer cells - Levy, J., et al. Nutrition & Cancer. 24(3):257-266, 1995.
28. Reduced death rate in women with breast cancer who performed regular exercise - JAMA 2005, May 25 293 pg 2479-86

REFERENCES

29. Bra wearing and the risk of developing breast cancer - Dressed to Kill by Soma Grismaijer, Sydney Ross Singer . Avery 1995
30. Bio-identical hormones - What your doctor may not tell you about menopause - by John R. Lee, M.D. and Virginia Hopkins Warner Books 2004
31. Meat intake and the risk of invasive prostate cancer - Gann et al, J nat Cancer institute 86; 1994, 281-86
32. Lycopene and prostate cancer - Ansari, M. S., et al. BJU. 92(4):375-378, 2003.
33. Melatonin and prostate cancer - Xi, S. C., et al Prostate. 46(1):52-61, 2001
34. Saw palmetto and prostate cancer - Iguchi, K., et al. Prostate. 47(1):59-65, 2001.
35. Multivitamin & selenium in reducing the risk of developing bowel cancer Ann Intern Med. 1998 Oct 1;129(7):517-24 and Clark L.C et al; JAMA. 1996 Dec 25;276(24):1957-63
36. Melatonin and bowel cancer - . Barni S, et al. Tumori. 1990;76:58-60.
37. Cimetidine and colorectal cancer survival Adams WJ, Morris DL. Lancet. 1994 Dec 24-31;344(8939-8940):1768-9
38. Cimetidine increases colorectal cancer patient survival - Matsumoto S, Imaeda Y, Umemoto S, Kobayashi K, Suzuki H, Okamoto T. Brit J Can 2002 (86) 161-167
39. Cimetidine and survival after gastric cancer - Tonnesen H, et al Lancet 1988 Oct 29;2(8618):990-2
40. Newcastle virus and stomach cancer - Csatary, L.; Cancer Detection and Prevention. Vol 17, N06, 1993. Pp. 619 - 627.
41. Melatonin and non small cell lung cancer - Lissoni, P., et al. Tunouri. 80(6):464-467, 1994.
42. Melatonin and melanoma – Reiter, Russel J. & Robinson, Jo. Melatonin. Bantam Books, New York, USA. 1996:98-100.
43. Astragalus may reduce the side effects of chemotherapy - Taixiang W. Munro AJ.et al Cochrane Database of Systematic Reviews. (1):CD004540, 2005
44. CoEnzyme Q10 and regression of breast cancer- Biochemical and biophysical research communication; vol. 199. No. 3, 1994 march 30, 1994 pages 1504 - 1508

REFERENCES

45. CoEnzyme Q10 and prostate cancer – normalization of PSA – William Judy (unpublished) http://www.newswithviews.com/Howenstine/james2.htm
46. CoQ10 causes cancer cells to self destruct - Lee et al. Ann NY Acad Sci.2005; 1042: 429-438
47. Garlic lowers the risk of developing cancers - Dorant E, et al. A critical review. Br J Cancer 1993;67:424–9
48. National Cancer Institute studies the value of Hydrazine in cancer. Review paper - http://www.nih.gov/news/pr/aug97/nci-19.htm
49. Dr Gold reviews the use of Hydrazine - http://www.hydrazinesulfate.org
50. Hyperthermia, National Cancer Institute review of hyperthermia - http://www.cancer.gov/cancertopics/factsheet/Therapy/hyperthermia
51. Indole 3 carbinol increases effectiveness of tamoxifen - Cover CM et a; I Cancer Res. 1999 Mar 15;59(6):1244-5
52. Laetrile – Sloan Kettering studies animal – discussion - http://www.curezone.com/diseases/cancer/laetrile.asp
53. Review of Lycopene and cancer - Giovannuccci E. - J Natl Cancer Inst 1999;91:317-31
54. Food and Drug Administration gives qualified support fro the preventive effects of Lycopene - http://www.cfsan.fda.gov/~dms/qhclyco2.html
55. Melatonin and cancer discussion - http://www.uni-koeln.de/symposium2000/contrib/index.html#5
56. Metformin reduces the incidence of pancreatic cancer in hamsters - http://www.cancerprev.org/Journal/Issues/26/101/1096/4412
57. Diabetic patients taking Metformin had 21% less cancer - Evans JMM, et al. BMJ 2005;330:1304-1305
58. Incidence of cancer related to selenium levels in the soil – review http://lpi.oregonstate.edu/f-w97/selenium.html
59. Selenium inhibits angiogenesis (blood vessel growth) in cancer - Mol Carcinogen 99, Vol. 26, Iss. 4, Pgs. 213-225
60. Turmeric may reduce resistance to chemotherapy - Chearwy W et al Cancer Chemother Pharmacol. 2006 Feb;57(3):376-88. Epub 2005 Jul 14
61. Turmeric may inhibit the effects of some chemotherapy -. Cancer Res. 2002 Jul 1;62(13):3868-75.
62. Turmeric as an anti-inflammatory to relieve pain - http://medherb.com/Materia_Medica/Curcuma_-_Turmeric_.htm

63. Depleted uranium – review - http://seattlepi.nwsource.com/national/95178_du12.shtml

64. Folic acid multivitamins reduce breast cancer in women who drink alcohol - Zhang S, Hunter DJ, Hankinson SE et al. JAMA 1999; 281:1632–7

65. Vitamin E reduces cancer in elderly people - KG Losonczy et al American Journal of Clinical Nutrition, Vol 64, 190-196

66. Fish oils reduce prostate cancer - Paul Terry et al; Lancet, 2nd June 2001

67. Oestrogen and progesterone imbalance - What Your Doctor May Not Tell You About Breast Cancer, by John R. Lee, MD, David Zava, PhD, and Virginia Hopkins, MA. Published by Warner Books 2002, New York, NY.

68. Breast cancer and age of first child – National Cancer Institute review - http://www.cancer.gov/cancertopics/factsheet/Risk/pregnancy

69. HRT increases the risk of breast cancer - January 26, 2000 Journal of the American Medical Association

70. Toxic compounds found in breast milk - http://www.health-report.co.uk/flame-retardant-toxic-chemicals.htm

71. Underarm deodorants - review from National Cancer Institute - http://www.cancer.gov/cancertopics/factsheet/Risk/AP-Deo

72. Parabens found in breast tumours - Darbre PD, , et al. Journal of Applied Toxicology 2004; 24:5–13

73. Future II trial on human papilovius vaccine for cervical cancer - Skjeldestad FE for the Future II steering committee Infectious Diseases Society of America, 43rd annual meeting San Francisco October 2005. Abstract LB-8a

74. How you can learn to meditate – Peace of Mind – Dr Ian Gawler Michelle Anderson Publishing 1999

75. Immune therapy and nasopharyngeal cancer - Comoli P, et al.. Journal of Clinical Oncology. October 3, 2005.

76. Immunological basis and immunotherapy of nasopharyngeal carcinoma. - Tsukuda M, Sawaki S.Auris Nasus Larynx. 1985;12 Suppl 2:S161-5

77. Destagnation herbs & radiotherapy in nasopharyngeal cancer - Xu, GZ et al Int. J. Radiation Oncology, Biol., and Physics (1989) 16:297.

INDEX

INDEX

INDEX

NOTES

NOTES

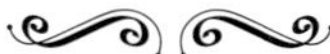

CANCER A Threat To Your Life? **or** A Chance To Control Your Future
First published 2006

Although the authors have researched many sources in the preparation of this book, they cannot take full responsibility for the accuracy and completeness of the information presented. Throughout the book we encourage people to discuss their treatment with their health professionals before undertaking any form of treatment.

OTHER BOOKS BY THE SAME AUTHORS:

Fad, Fable or fact – Dietary Supplements, the scientific documentation about our diet and the use of dietary supplements.

Fad, Fable or fact – Coronary Heart Disease, a review of all the treatments available.

Enquiries – glewis@clear.net.nz

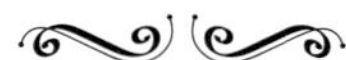